manuka

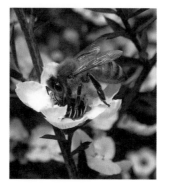

manuka

the biography of an extraordinary HONEY

CLIFF VAN EATON

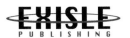

EXISLE PUBLISHING

First published 2014

Exisle Publishing Limited,
P.O. Box 60-490, Titirangi, Auckland 0642, New Zealand.
'Moonrising', Narone Creek Road, Wollombi, NSW 2325, Australia.
www.exislepublishing.com

A catalogue record for this book is available from the National Library of
New Zealand.

ISBN 978-1-77559-163-4

10 9 8 7 6 5 4 3 2 1

Disclaimer: This book is a general guide only and should never be a
substitute for the skill, knowledge, and experience of a qualified medical
professional dealing with the facts, circumstances and symptoms of a
particular case. The author and the publisher are not responsible for any
adverse effects or consequences resulting from the use of the information
in this book. It is the responsibility of the reader to consult a physician
or other qualified healthcare professional regarding his or her personal
health. The book contains references to products that may not be available
everywhere. The intent of the information provided is to be helpful;
however, there is no guarantee of results associated with the information
provided. Use of brand names does not imply endorsement.

Cover and text design and production by Art Rowlands
Printed in Shenzhen, China, by Ink Asia

To Peter Molan

An immigrant scientist and non-beekeeper
who has had the greatest impact on New Zealand beekeeping
since Mary Bumby arrived with the first two skeps
of honey bees in 1839

CONTENTS

ACKNOWLEDGEMENTS

In researching this project, I have been able to call on my own experiences in New Zealand as a beekeeping advisor, bee disease specialist, consultant and scientist over 30 years. I've been extremely fortunate to be able to watch the story of manuka honey as it has unfolded over almost that entire time, and I have even had a few direct personal experiences with the honey, both when nobody seemed to want it, and when it developed into one of the most famous (and certainly most expensive) honeys in the world.

More than that, however, I have been helped beyond measure by a number of people who have played central roles in the whole saga. In particular I want to give a special vote of thanks to Dr Peter Molan, who so kindly agreed to a very long interview, as well as provided thoughtful answers to my numerous email queries. Full of energy, ever-inquisitive, and a great communicator of often complicated science in a way that manages to excite the rest of us, Peter is undoubtedly the star of this book.

Thanks also go to the following people for agreeing to interviews: Kerry Simpson, Murray Reid, Malcolm Haines, Les Blackwell, Bill Floyd, Bill Bracks, Julie Betts, Dr Jonathan Stephens and Dr Ralf Schlothauer. They are all important characters whom you will meet in the pages to come, and the time they spent with me sharing their recollections and insights was the most rewarding part of the whole book-writing experience.

After all these years Alan Bougen remains a close personal friend, and he has been my most constant source of encouragement throughout the process of researching, composing and editing this book. My former colleague Dr Mark Goodwin kindly offered access to the archives at Ruakura Agricultural Research Centre, without doubt the most extensive source of historical beekeeping material in New Zealand. And Murray Reid, a fellow beekeeping advisor for many years, opened his 'ark-hives' to me as well. To all three of these great mates, cheers!

Thanks also must go to Bogdan Gan, at Kiwi Bee Ltd, for showing me the company's extraction and processing facility for medical-grade manuka honey, the most technologically sophisticated 'beekeeper's shed' I have ever seen. And *kia ora* to Kuini Puru of the New Zealand Historic Places Trust for coming in on her day off to take me through the mission house at Mangungu.

I am extremely grateful to Gareth St John Thomas and his team at Exisle Publishing, who have been so supportive in allowing me to write this 'different sort of book' on honey. Ian Watt has been a calm and steady influence during the entire book-making process, including book design and proof-reading.

Lastly, let me beg one further moment of your time to pay tribute to my dear Bonnie — best friend, life-partner, and chief cook and bottle-washer these past months. Hugs beyond measure, and kisses sweeter than honey!

A note on using this book

As I hope will become clear, this is not a scholarly book, and it therefore doesn't include those little note numbers in the text which you often find sprinkled through scientific works, corresponding to an imposing set of bibliographic references. The book does, however, contain a number of interesting facts and challenging ideas, and so a Notes section has been included at the end of the book to provide more information about the sources I have used. The Notes section is divided by chapter, and each note begins with the referring page number. As well, in the text itself you will sometimes find an asterisk (*) symbol. This indicates that there is more information about the topic being discussed in the Notes at the end of the book.

A QUICK INTRODUCTION

The book you are about to read is not a comprehensive scholarly review of manuka honey, or even of honey in general. There are other publications that attempt to do the latter, not to mention the well over 2500 scientific papers just on the therapeutic properties of manuka honey alone. Those sorts of works can certainly be useful, if sometimes hard for the layman to understand. But the real problem is that, unless you are very good at reading between the lines, they leave out much of what is a very remarkable story indeed.

This book is something a bit different: a biography, but not of the usual sort. There are plenty of human characters in the pages that follow, but the subject of this biography is actually a substance, and a very extraordinary one at that. It's a rags-to-riches tale of how a most peculiar honey became a ground-breaking medicine, along the way turning into one of the most famous honeys in the world. Not so long ago beekeepers literally gave the stuff away. Today you can find manuka honey almost everywhere, from a traditional Chinese medicine dispensary in Shanghai to a children's burn clinic in Baghdad; and from hospital wards in Great Britain to a stylish specialty food emporium in Rome.

Manuka is a word that the great Polynesian voyagers, the Maori, gave to a plant they discovered when they first came to the islands they called Aotearoa. Hundreds of years later, when Europeans brought honey bees to that same country now known as New Zealand, the bees began producing a very different sort of honey from that plant.

The honey was hard to get out of the combs, and even harder for beekeepers to sell. But eventually an inquisitive university lecturer discovered that it had a unique property, one that had never been found in honey before. And it soon became apparent that the honey could successfully treat wounds that didn't heal any other way. As a result, today the words manuka honey have become firmly established in the world's vocabulary, as well-known a New Zealand icon as kiwifruit. The pages that follow tell the story of how it got that way.

This is a book intended for the general reader. In fact, anyone with even a casual curiosity about manuka honey should, I hope, enjoy it. It hasn't been written specifically for beekeepers, although they may find something of interest, rather than instruction, in its pages. And it is hopefully free of science-based jargon. In the past I may have been a technical writer, but I know above all else that specialists who aren't able to communicate their knowledge in a way that the rest of the world can understand aren't really doing their job.

Instead, my intention has been to tell what is known in New Zealand as 'a good Kiwi yarn'. It is by turns part history (natural and human), part biology, and part scientific discovery. There's even a smattering of economics, as well as a bit of philosophy thrown in for good measure. But, above all else, this is a story of hope for the future; a piece of optimism in a world that for good reason feels saddened and sometimes even afraid about the future of a special relationship we humans have always had with those marvellous creatures, the honey bees. To learn about the good news, however, you'll have to read the book all the way to the end!

Cliff Van Eaton
April 2014

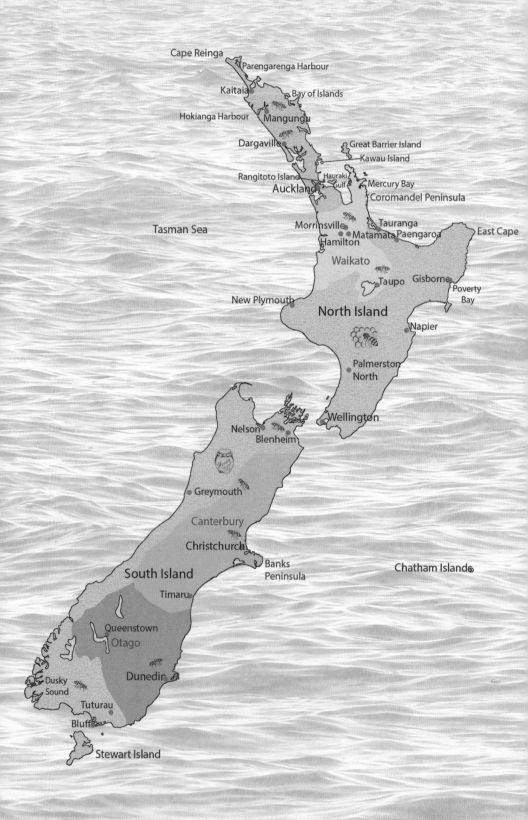

One

THE SAMPLE THAT DIDN'T MAKE SENSE

Peter Molan had a problem. There was his job at the University of Waikato, of course, teaching students the intricacies of biochemistry, the science of the compounds and chemical processes that make up living things. As well, he had taken on quite a bit of research. He was contracted three days a week to a local diary factory, helping them work out how to extract some special substances from cow's milk. And scientists at two of the local agricultural research institutes had also asked for his help in determining just what was responsible for a rather strange discovery they had made, namely that bull semen (of all things) was able to kill bacteria.

But while all that work certainly kept him busy, the problem concerned something else entirely. There was this small experiment, testing some local honeys against bacteria, which he had let a high-school teacher carry out in his lab over the summer holidays in January 1980 … and one of the samples just didn't make sense. The teacher had then gone off to a new job with the then Ministry of Agriculture. But the little mystery remained. And Peter being Peter, he just couldn't let it go. So now he was going to have to follow his own edict, the thing he always said when students came to him with a seemingly unexpected result: 'do the test again'.

Peter didn't know the first thing about honey, let alone the honeys produced in New Zealand, and for a very good reason. He came from industrialised Great Britain, half a world away. The reason he had ended up in Hamilton, New Zealand, in the heart of an area called the Waikato, with some of the best pasture-based dairy land in the world, at a university with a fairly new School

Opposite New Zealand, the home of manuka honey.

of Science, was the same as for many people who have come to the country over the generations — he wanted a safe, uncrowded, unspoiled place to raise a family.

A World War II baby, Peter was born in Cardiff, and spent a fair amount of his first year of life being taken in and out of a bomb shelter, since his mother's family home was near an armaments factory, the sort of place that was a popular target for German bombing raids.

His father, who was serving with the British forces, managed a very short leave to see his first-born, before heading back for training that culminated in his being wounded when his Sherman tank was shelled on the beach during the D-Day invasion in Normandy.

Peter's childhood was also spent in that Welsh city, a gritty harbour terminus for coal trains, no doubt made worse by the deprivation that accompanied post-war rationing throughout Britain. But while his upbringing was typically working class, it was his good fortune to go to a primary school with teachers who, as he says, 'got their pupils' brains working hard'. And his parents were equally supportive, not even getting angry when their energetic and inquisitive young son took their old-fashioned alarm clock to bits. As Peter says, that created an urge to find out how things worked, an urge that has never left him.

He also successfully made his way through the dreaded 11-plus exams, which streamed young people in Britain towards either manual training and the trades, or preparation for university and professional careers. He did so well in these tests, in fact, that he secured a place in the leading state grammar school in the city, an institution on a par with the fee-paying private schools that are normally the reserve of the wealthy and well-connected. It was his high-school teachers who showed him just how interesting science could be.

There followed an undergraduate degree in biochemistry at the local university (where his first child was born just before his final, third-year exams), and then a PhD in Liverpool, since the university there was offering a paying position that he could use to help support his wife and child. But when he completed his doctorate (studying the way saliva stimulated bacteria to produce acid in the mouth), he started looking for a teaching position overseas. Every week he would take out some books on different countries from the library, and one day he saw a job advertised for a lecturer at a university in the North Island of New Zealand. The pictures in the books made the country look like just the sort of place they wanted to live, especially compared with the still bombed-out parts of hard-bitten Liverpool. And so, after being accepted for the job without even an interview, Peter and his young family headed off to the Antipodes.

When he arrived at the university, the laboratory building had just been built. It was so new, in fact, that the window blinds hadn't been installed, and he spent his first summer setting up the labs with newspapers sellotaped to the windows to keep out the heat and glare.

It was an exciting time and, while student numbers were still low, the university was keen to recruit the best and the brightest from high schools throughout the region. So an out-reach programme was started, with lecturers visiting schools to demonstrate simple experiments and interact with staff. Peter really enjoyed the challenge. Being young himself, and certainly energetic, he also had a gift of being able to explain difficult concepts in a simple and easy-to-understand way. And so he took himself off to Otorohanga College, a high school 50 kilometres south of Hamilton in a small rural servicing town.

It was on one of those outings that he met Kerry Simpson, and formed a friendship that would change his life. Kerry was also from Britain, and had come to New Zealand for much the same reason as Peter. But Kerry also had an interest (or, as he would call it, 'a fascination') with bees. It had started when as a child he saw a Colonel Blimp-like character in moustache and tweeds moving rather animatedly through a field with a butterfly net. Kerry couldn't help himself: he just had to talk to the man, who turned out to be one of those wonderful gifts to the world of science that the English seem to produce in abundance — the talented (and obsessed) amateur. He was an expert in bee species, and took quite a bit of time explaining to the young boy their names and habits. After that, insects flying by were no longer just bugs to Kerry, and as time went on and he studied biology at university, he began to dream of one day having a beehive or two (and a back garden big enough to keep them in). He finally got his wish, after moving to New Zealand and eventually taking on the job as head of science at the high school in Otorohanga.

Peter and Kerry enjoyed each other's company, and on several occasions their families socialised together. So Peter's lab at the university was a natural choice when Kerry needed somewhere to carry out a little experiment. He had decided to become an Apicultural Advisory Officer with the Ministry of Agriculture, and his initial training was taking place nearby. He was going to trade teaching students for helping beekeepers with their problems, but before he could begin he needed to complete some sort of research project to do with honey bees. Kerry had read that honey was supposed to be antibacterial, and someone had told him that one particular variety, produced from a New Zealand native shrub called manuka, was very good for treating cuts and burns. So he thought he would test that honey, along with a couple of others (blackberry and clover) that he had collected from his own hives.

There was nothing very complicated about the experiment. In fact, the basics go back to the 1880s when Robert Koch, a German physician, discovered how to grow (or *culture*) bacteria on thin, circular glass dishes developed by his friend Julius Petri. As a material (or *media*) on which to grow the bacteria, he first tried potatoes, but eventually settled on agar, a gelatine made from a certain type of seaweed.* Koch used these Petri dishes (or *plates*) to good effect, isolating a species of *Bacillus* bacteria (which he was able to grow on the plate as a pure culture), and then showing, to the acclaim of the world, that it was the cause of tuberculosis. The plates, the culturing methods, and the requirements needed to prove that an organism causes a disease (called 'Koch's Postulates') are still in widespread use today.

Louis Pasteur had used a similar type of culturing method in the 1860s to show that heating beer, wine and milk killed the bacteria that often spoiled them (a process the world thanked him for by calling it *pasteurisation*). And Paul Ehrlich also employed it at the turn of the next century in developing the concept of chemotherapy for the treatment of disease, with a compound that was a remarkably effective treatment for syphilis (and in so doing coining the term 'magic bullet').* But culturing bacteria was perfected by Alexander

Fleming, and in fact it was an old agar plate of *Staphylococcus* bacteria overgrown with bread mould that led to his discovery in 1928 of the first and most famous antibiotic of all time, penicillin.*

It's a very small world

We should now pause for a moment and say a few words about some important fellow inhabitants of this planet where we reside. Microbes are everywhere in our world. Or, as Bill Bryson puts it much more correctly in *A Short History of Nearly Everything*, we are just a small part of *theirs*.* It sounds absurd, but when it comes to living things the tiny are a lot bigger than the rest. Those divisions of life smaller than our eyes can see make up way more of what's around us than all the other plants and animals put together. Individually we may not be able to see them, but together microbes have four times more biomass. The reason we often don't notice them is that so many live underground. Again, as Bryson says, if you took all of the bacteria out of the Earth's interior and dumped them on the surface, they would cover everything to the height of a four-storey building.

Without microbes we literally wouldn't exist. We may thank bigger organisms like plants for supplying us with some of the oxygen we breathe, but algae and other microbes produce far more. And without bacteria grabbing nitrogen from the atmosphere and turning it into organic molecules called nucleotides and amino acids, no larger creatures could survive.

As for our up-close-and-personal relationship with bacteria, while they may be single-celled organisms, on a cell-for-cell basis there are 10 times more of them on us and in us than there are human cells that make up our body. Most of them are very useful, especially in helping us digest the food we eat. But among them are also many dangerous species, ones that often cause devastating epidemics and much else. So one of the great turning points in human history has to have been when we finally worked out that 'germs' like bacteria could be the cause of illness. It's something that these days we just take for granted, as if we've always known it was true. But amazingly we have had telephones and lights in our homes for about the same amount of time as we have known for certain that bacteria were the cause of many diseases. Before that, even the greatest minds were apt to blame 'bad air' for cholera, and 'being too clean' for the plague.*

But while disease-causing microbes are everywhere, both animals and plants are also excellent at working out ways of dealing with these intruders, using molecules produced internally, along with an array of cells and cell processes (although those activities in our own immune system can often make us feel very unwell).

We humans are also ingenuous, and so we have worked out ways of dealing to many of the microbes that might harm us by coming up with compounds that either work directly on the microbes themselves, or stimulate our immune system to work more effectively against them. And of course many of these compounds originate from nature, even though we have become very good at making them in the laboratory as well. It is in these natural compounds, however, that we get some understanding of how the immune systems of plants work against microbes, and also how those plant substances can do many of the same things when we consume them or apply them to ourselves.

Natural products have been a particularly rich source of antibiotics, yielding, for example, the penicillins (from Fleming's bread mould) in 1940, the tetracyclines (from soil bacteria) in 1948, and the glycopeptides, including antibiotics such as vancomycin (from another soil bacteria, in 1953).

To study the effect is a fairly simple matter of putting a small amount of a known species or strain of bacteria into a sterile dish together with some nutrient for the bacteria to live on. Next you add to the plate the substance that you want to test, incubate the plate for a while, and then measure the *inhibition ring* (the area around the substance where the bacteria didn't grow).

And that's what Kerry and Peter did with honey, a plant product altered by bees that humans were using as a healing substance thousands of years before we ever figured out that bacteria caused disease. The only twist they made came about because of some reading Peter had done. Honey produces hydrogen peroxide when it is diluted, and in 1962 it was shown that this made the honey antibacterial. But Peter also found a few scientific papers that mentioned other, non-peroxide activities of some honeys. So Peter and Kerry hit on the idea of knocking out the hydrogen peroxide, using an enzyme that is present in all living organisms called *catalase*.

The experiment took only a couple of days, although they had to wait for the bacterial cultures to grow, and for the honey to stop the bacteria in its tracks. All three honeys created a circle of inhibition when the catalase wasn't used. But once the hydrogen peroxide was eliminated, both the blackberry and clover honeys had no effect. The other honey, on the other hand, the one produced by bees collecting nectar from the manuka shrub, really dealt to the bacteria. As Kerry said, 'It was only one sample, but it still had this astonishing activity. Manuka was the winner, hands down.'

Testing the weeds

Kerry Simpson didn't think anything more about his little experiment. He recalls writing down the results in a standard school exercise book, and he can even remember drawing some graphs. But he had other things on his mind, like trying to pack as much beekeeping information into his head as he could before he went further south to take up his first position with the Ministry. Years later, when manuka honey became famous, he went looking for the notebooks again. But in his family's numerous moves (including living in the tiny Pacific island nation of Tuvalu), the papers had been lost.*

In Peter's case, however, it was quite the opposite. It was like that clock his parents had let him take apart as a child. He just had to figure out what was going on with that one honey. The only way to know for sure whether the test was in error was to collect a lot more samples — not just of manuka, but of a whole host of other New Zealand-produced honeys as well — and see what happened.

Luckily he had a lot of help. There was a graduate student, Kate Russell, who needed a topic for her master's degree. And there were two technicians, Mary Smith and Kerry Allen, who helped run the labs where students did the practical work that complemented the lectures they received. They needn't have got involved, but they were just as interested as Peter, and they had more training in the disciplines of bacterial cultures and *diffusion assays* (the way the bacterial inhibition created by an antibacterial substance is tested and measured). Peter was a biochemist, not a microbiologist, after all.

He also had a friend who could probably get him some honey samples. Murray Reid had helped train Kerry Simpson as a bee-keeping advisor in the Ministry of Agriculture, and he was stationed nearby in Hamilton. He knew a lot of beekeepers, and also had colleagues around the country with similar contacts. So Murray put out the word, and eventually a large number of honey samples began arriving at Peter's lab.

There was white clover (*Trifolium repens*), of course, the most popular honey in the country, and the one most often produced by beekeepers, since the plant was spread throughout New Zealand's pastures, and helped make them bountiful by fixing nitrogen into the soil. There were also a few samples of buttercup (*Ranunculus repens*), a spring species associated with wet pastures, as well as a number of samples marked simply as 'mixed pasture', since the colour of the honey was darker than the normally very white of clover honey, and it had a slightly stronger taste as well. All sorts of species might have contributed nectar to the final honey produced by the bees, including the so-called yellow weeds like cat's ear (*Hypochaeris radicata*) that sprout up in summer once the pasture begins to dry out.

Many of the other samples came from what could quite rightly be called herbs, although in the New Zealand context they weren't just coming from a couple of plants in someone's garden. These were species that may originally have been brought to the country for culinary or medicinal purposes, but which liked the local environment so much that they established themselves as wild escapees, in some cases even becoming what the authorities now called 'noxious weeds'. Among them was penny royal (*Mentha pulegium*), a low-growing plant that literally hides in pasture, but which gives itself away when it's walked over since it has such a strong, minty fragrance. The honey is fairly dark and, while it is distinctive, it doesn't taste of mint at all.

And then there was thyme (*Thymus vulgaris*). It is said that this famous Mediterranean herb was planted in the garden of a large farm in the South Island (called a 'sheep station'), since it was a very nice addition to roast lamb. But the plant found the environment in a particular part of Central Otago, along the dry rocks cut into canyons by the mighty Clutha River, to be so perfect that

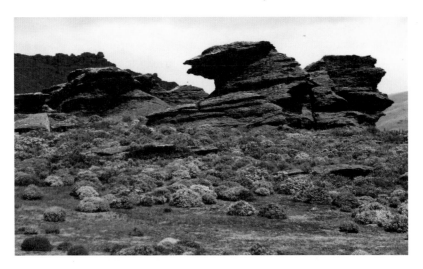

Thyme (*Thymus vulgaris*), the garden escapee that now covers the rock canyons of the mighty Clutha River in Central Otago.

in no time it had displaced almost every other growing thing in the area, turning the steep cliffs and high flats a wondrous purple hue in the spring. Like penny royal, the ankle-deep thyme plants give off an aroma that is almost overpowering when you walk among them. The honey, of medium amber colour, tastes — at least to some people — the way Chinese incense smells.*

A final herb provided a further half-dozen samples of honey, but this one wasn't a fugitive, at least not at the beginning of its existence in New Zealand. Heather (*Calluna vulgaris*) is well known to anyone who has walked the Highlands of Scotland, and fondness for home is probably what led some enterprising developers (and the government, it must be said) to plant it around the base of the volcanic mountains in the central North Island of New Zealand in the early 1900s in the country's first national park.

The heather was meant to go along with the grouse they hoped to release as part of a plan to encourage well-heeled tourists to spend a shooting holiday in these newly created Antipodean Highlands, complete with a stay in a grand house in the European tradition called The Chateau. The grouse never eventuated, although The Chateau still stands, and, while honey bees clearly love the plant (and people in Europe love the honey the bees produce from it), heather in New Zealand is now officially another noxious plant.*

Honeys like no others

Along with these introduced weeds (and for honey bees, finding what we call 'weeds' spread all over the countryside is their version of paradise), Peter Molan and his team also received a number of honey samples that were unique to New Zealand. Cut off from the rest of the world for tens of millions of years, the ecosystems of the North and South Islands developed a wide range of flowering trees and shrubs, many of which produced enough nectar to provide at least partially for the food needs of some species of birds. In fact, when the flowers bloomed there was so much nectar that, once European settlers arrived, the honey bees they brought with them produced large crops of a number of honey varieties, many of which had never been seen before anywhere else in the world.

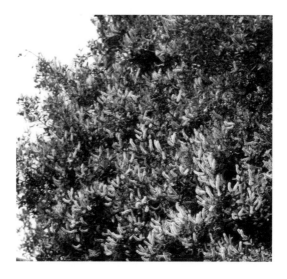

Kamahi (*Weinmannia racemosa*), the tree that produces a distinctive-tasting honey often blended with other honeys to make 'bush blend'.

In the samples there was the dark, flavoursome honey from rewarewa (*Knightia excelsa*), a tall, straight tree with reddish tube-shaped flowers common in the redeveloping forest margins in parts of the North Island. There was also tawari (*Ixerba brexioides*), a unique, bushy tree with shiny green leaves and bright white flowers that grows only in a couple of select ranges around Auckland and the Bay of Plenty, and which for some reason doesn't lend itself to planting in garden landscapes. And there was kamahi (*Weinmannia racemosa*), a medium-sized forest tree that grows in both the North and South Islands, and its close cousin towai (*Weinmannia silvicola*), from the northern parts of the North Island. The honey itself is of a light yellow colour, with a taste that New Zealanders have long been accustomed to since it always makes up a fair portion of what beekeepers sell as 'bush blend'. There were even a couple of samples of honey from rata, including the forest giant *Metrosideros umbellata* that looms over the rain forest of the South Island's west coast with its bright red flowers, and the far more diminutive vine rata (*Metrosideros perforata*), that climbs trees in the North Island bush.

Finally, there was manuka (*Leptospermum scoparium*), and with it a couple of samples of its close relative called kanuka (once named *Leptospermum ericoides* by the botanists, but these days now included in the Kunzeas as *Kunzea ericoides*). Beekeepers had a hard time selling honeys from these two species, and the honey itself was difficult to remove from the combs. It was a peculiar honey that not very many people wanted but, as Kerry found with his original single sample, it was nevertheless intriguing — and produced results that just didn't make sense.

Hydrogen peroxide, osmosis, and sweet and sour

The many honeys Peter Molan and his team tested in the lab were diluted with water until they made up only 25% of the total solution, then droplets were put into small holes (*wells*) cut into the agar in the Petri dish. The agar itself contained the bacteria *Staphylococcus aureus*, an organism routinely used in tests of antibacterial activity. *S. aureus* — or staph, as it is more commonly known — is found in both the human respiratory tract and on the skin, and is the cause of both chest infections and boils. It has an even nastier side, however, since it is very adept at developing resistance to man-made antibiotics, and creates infections in over half a million patients in American hospitals each year.

S. aureus also produces catalase, but Peter and the team added more of the enzyme to destroy any hydrogen peroxide the honey may have produced, just as Peter and Kerry had done in the original experiment.

But hydrogen peroxide isn't the only way honey kills bacteria. It is also highly acidic, with a pH (a measure of how acid or alkaline a substance is) about the same as weak vinegar. Most bacteria prefer a pH of between 7.2 to 7.4 for optimum growth, whereas the normal range in honey is 3.2 to 4.5. In fact, it is often said that if honey wasn't so sweet it would really be sour. And it is that sweetness which gives honey its other major ability to keep bacteria at bay.

Honey is what is called a 'super-saturated' sugar solution, with a moisture level that can vary, but when sealed in honey comb (or a jar) is generally below 20%. It's 'super' because if we try to just dissolve sugar in water we can't get below 36% moisture (or to put it the other way, above 64° *brix*, the number of grams of sugar in 100 ml of solution), which is the solution's natural equilibrium. What that means in practical terms is that when honey is exposed to the atmosphere (or bacteria) it attracts moisture to itself, trying to reach that equilibrium. It acts almost like a sponge, and literally sucks the life out microbes that are exposed to it. It's what chemists refer to as *osmosis*, the passage of molecules in a liquid, through a membrane, to an area outside that isn't as dilute, until the dilutions are equal. It's the way water moves into and out of the cells of all living things.

Only spores of a select few species of bacteria (especially one causing a serious bee disease) and fungi (the ones that turn dilute honey into mead) with really hard protein coats can withstand this *osmotic pressure*, the spores waiting for a time when the sugar/water solution making up the honey becomes dilute enough that the fungi can germinate. For Peter and his tests, *S. aureus* proved to be a perfect organism in this regard, because it isn't affected by either the acidity of the honey or its high sugar concentration. It can be a tough bacteria to kill.*

In these first tests, most of the honeys managed to inhibit the growth of the *S. aureus* on the plate, at least a bit. But the area cleared of bacterial growth was much larger for many of the manuka and kanuka samples, along with a couple of samples of penny royal and a pasture weed common in the Hawke's Bay region called nodding thistle. Other samples of nodding thistle honey didn't produce any activity against the bacteria, however. So that one sample of manuka honey in Kerry Simpson's first experiment clearly wasn't a fluke. Not every sample had the same level of activity, however, and there was the suggestion that in at least a few of the samples there was the possibility of misidentification, since all they had to go on was the name written on the container, and with it presumably the experience of the beekeeper who supplied it.

A sample of manuka was also provided by Murray Reid from his own resources. It was a little 25-gram gift jar of honey that Air New Zealand had long ago provided to its business and first-class international passengers to spread on their in-flight toast at breakfast. Murray had kept it in a cupboard at work for years, but gave it to Peter to test thinking that it would provide a perfect control, since it wouldn't be likely to have any antibacterial action, hydrogen peroxide-based or otherwise. The honey was almost completely black in colour, but to everyone's surprise it had one of the highest levels of activity in the test, a result which, as we will see in a subsequent chapter of this book, only made sense years later.

More tests were then carried out on the manuka and kanuka honeys. Samples were heated to 95° Celsius for over an hour, and yet they still killed the bacteria. The honey was also diluted with water twenty-fold, and tested against a much greater variety of bacteria. Only 3 of the 12 species weren't affected. Clearly, the antibacterial activity of the manuka and kanuka honey samples was very unusual, and also very strong.

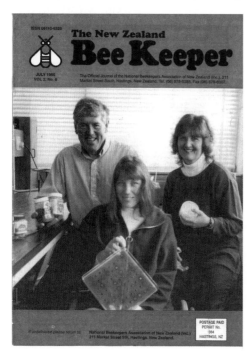

Peter Molan, Nicolette Brady and Kerry Allen, in the University of Waikato lab where much of the early work on manuka honey took place.

'Absolutely no interest to anybody'

As any scientist will tell you, just because you find something unusual in an experiment doesn't mean that everyone else is going to think your effort has been worthwhile. Based on this first collection of 64 honey samples from around the country, Kate Russell was at least able to write up some of the testing for her Master's of Science thesis.*

Peter himself felt the results were sufficiently worthwhile to share with the wider world in the form of a scientific paper. However, when he submitted his first paper to the *New Zealand Journal of Agricultural Research*, he was shocked by the reply from the editor, which Peter remembers as stating quite bluntly 'The topic of this paper is of absolutely no interest to anybody.' Thankfully other journals overseas didn't display quite such an unfortunate attitude, and two papers describing the work finally appeared in the *Journal of Apicultural Research*, at the time the world's most important review of beekeeping science. The first, by Peter, Mary Smith and Murray Reid, showed that the antibacterial activity of manuka honey was significantly higher than that of clover and heather honeys, but concluded that many more samples would need to be tested to determine the relative activities of all the various honeys.* The second, written by Peter and Kate Russell, described the *nonperoxide activity* (a term that would eventually be abbreviated as NPA by scientists and beekeepers alike) found in some honeys, which they concluded was not due to other factors like acidity and sugar concentration, and which was linked to floral origin.*

Work continued in the lab, as time and resources permitted, still being fitted in amidst the teaching and the dairy research. Finally in 1991 another paper was published, this time in a well-known international journal published by the Pharmaceutical Society of Great Britain. Scientists from outside the country were now beginning to take an interest in the antibacterial activities of some New Zealand honeys, and in fields in addition to *apiculture* (the science of beekeeping).*

A much larger number of honey samples had now been tested (345 to be exact, although 79 were not identified to floral source by the beekeepers who provided them). Of that total, 50 were stated to be manuka, and a further 20 were kanuka. Catalase was again added to the samples to remove the hydrogen peroxide. And crucially, a system that was standard to all types of antibacterial testing was employed not just to measure the inhibition ring in the bacterial culture created by the adding of honey to the test well, but also to compare the inhibition to the concentration of phenol. The system was a modification of an assay for antibacterial substances used in the New Zealand dairy industry, something Kerry Allen was quite used to, and which together with Peter she helped modify for use with honey.

10+, 15+, 20+

Phenol, otherwise known as carbolic acid, was first extracted from coal tar in the early part of the nineteenth century, and was used by Joseph Lister, beginning in 1867, in his pioneering development of antiseptic methods of surgery. Since then countless children have also come into contact with it, since it is the active ingredient in carbolic soap. In the tests of New Zealand honey, it provided the all-important comparative standard.

In the test assay, plates much larger than the old Petri dishes were used, and they were square, not round. In each plate, a total of 64 wells were punched, and honey samples were placed at random in the wells, both with and without catalase. The clear zone (the inhibition ring) was measured in millimetres using callipers.

The result was then compared with that from another plate where concentrations of phenol were put in wells, and the circle where the bacteria wouldn't grow was measured. The higher the *phenol equivalent*, the stronger the antibacterial activity of the honey, since the honey created an inhibition zone similar to a higher concentration of phenol.

Non-peroxide activity was only found in samples of honey from manuka, as well as a few from viper's bugloss, another plant introduced into the dry areas of the South Island from Australia, where it had traditionally been used as a drought-resistant species suitable for sheep. The viper's bugloss results weren't all that spectacular. Only four samples showed activity, and the average was equivalent to about 4% phenol (similar to the concentration that was used in some less irritating brands of that old-fashioned carbolic soap). The manuka honey, on the other hand, showed non-peroxide

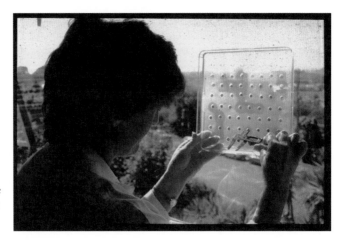

Kerry Allen, Peter Molan's long-time collaborator and assistant, measuring manuka honey's circle of bacterial inhibition with callipers.

activity levels that were on average about four and a half times that level, with activity typically equivalent to 15–30% phenol. One sample even tested out at a whopping 58% phenol equivalent. And the use of catalase, as well as the comparisons made on the much bigger plates, showed pretty conclusively that the antibacterial activity was in many cases almost entirely caused by something in the honey other than hydrogen peroxide.

The testing also made much clearer an observation that was perhaps apparent in the previous work, but which couldn't be concluded with certainty because of the smaller number of samples involved: there were significant differences in non-peroxide antibacterial activity in manuka honey samples supplied by beekeepers from around the country. In fact, only about 40% showed this sort of activity.

This study, the results of which were published by Peter Molan and Kerry Allen, provided for the first time a means of measuring the non-peroxide antibacterial activity of manuka honey in a way that could readily be understood by the general public, and it would become established in the years to come as a rating system on manuka honey products sold for therapeutic products (the well-known 10+, 15+ and 20+). It was certainly needed, because it was now obvious that not all manuka honey was created equal.

But big questions still remained. What was causing these differences in activity? And, even more fundamentally (because Peter still had his parents' alarm clock firmly fixed in his mind), what was the 'magic ingredient' that was so special (perhaps unique) in this one honey only really produced in New Zealand?

Most of all, however, how could the discovery of this different sort of antibacterial activity, and the honey that produced it, be put to any sort of practical use?

The answers to these questions, and the way manuka honey went from a neglected food product to a mainstream medicine, is what most of the rest of this book is about. But before we begin, let's go back to basics and learn a bit more about those fascinating and sometimes frightening creatures, the honey bees. After all, if bees hadn't produced a food from the nectar they collected from manuka flowers, we may never have discovered what an amazing substance manuka honey truly is. It's just another example of our species-long relationship with these remarkable insects, one that we are only just learning to fully appreciate now that it is so very much in jeopardy.

Two

YOU NEVER
CAN TELL
WITH BEES[†]

A celebrated study on the use of tools by primates describes a chimpanzee, the animal species closest to us genetically, using a stick to probe into a wild bee nest to extract honey. No one knows, of course, how long humans have had an association with honey bees, but given the dexterity of that chimp, it is probably safe to say that it's been for a very long time.

The earliest surviving human record of that connection isn't on some ancient papyrus, however. It instead appears on a cliff face, since it pre-dates the invention of writing by about 3000 years. A rock painting in the La Araña cave in Bicorp, Spain, depicts a person with fairly wide hips and longish hair (known for some reason as the *Man* of Bicorp) clinging onto what is believed to be wild grape or clematis vines, with honey bees flying all around. The 'man' is reaching into the nest with one hand, and grasping a basket with the other, no doubt to hold the spoils. Far below, a much thinner helper with another container on his/her back is climbing up to help. The obviously brave collectors were immortalised on the wall about 8000 years ago, not very long after the end of the last Ice Age, at a time when the region was enjoying a particularly

---

[†] Honey bees are probably the most studied of all insects. But while we have been able to unlock a number of their secrets, there is still very much we have to learn. So as beekeepers and scientists alike will tell you, the title of this chapter is one of the most profound things ever said about honey bees. The author of the quote isn't a Nobel Prize winner, however, although everyone knows him nevertheless. He's the world's most famous honey specialist — Winnie-the-Pooh!

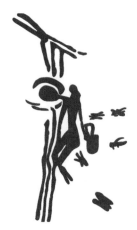

The Man of Bicorp, the earliest surviving human record of our long association with honey bees.

good climate. But rest assured, this wasn't an isolated occurrence. Similar depictions can be found in both southern Africa and India, and as anyone can attest who has watched television documentaries on the modern-day honey hunters in Malaysia and Nepal, the practice is still going on today in some parts of the world.

The first representation we have of actual bee 'keeping', on the other hand, dates from about 2500 BC, in Ancient Egypt. Part of a bas-relief on an Egyptian sun temple in the lower Nile shows honey being collected from hives. Even though the carving is much deteriorated, a kneeling man can still be seen blowing smoke through a vessel (the first recorded 'bee smoker') onto a stack of six cylinders. Three other people are putting the harvested honey into big clay jars.

A more complete depiction, however, in the form of a wall painting, can be found high up in the corner of the tomb of Rekhmire in Luxor, Egypt, dating from a thousand years later. Here there can be no doubt about what is going on. One worker uses a very sophisticated smoker, while the other removes combs of honey and places them into two bowls. There are even a couple of smudges of what look like bees flying in the air. And the beekeepers are almost as brave as the Bicorp honey hunters. They seem to be wearing nothing more than loincloths.

The earliest known written record, on the other hand, comes from a set of Hittite laws inscribed on a clay tablet in about 1500 BC, which were found in Anatolia, 1000 kilometres to the north. They set out the revised fines to be paid if someone stole hives, either empty or occupied by bees. Formerly it was a pound of silver for a swarm, and exposure to bee stings for two or three hives (ouch!). The new fines were only five or six shekels, but your house was held as a guarantee that you paid.*

Beekeeping was certainly thriving in the ancient kingdom, since another record shows that Ramses III (1186–1155 BC) made an offering of 20 tonnes of honey to the gods. That's a lot, even by

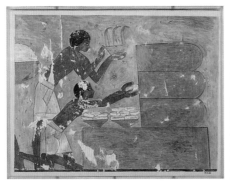

A wall painting from the tomb of Rekhmire around 1500 BC, showing beekeepers in loincloths using a smoker to help harvest honey from their hives. Beekeeping was highly advanced in ancient Egypt, and beehives were even transported down the Nile on barges.

today's standards, and would have represented the harvest from at least 5000 clay hives.*

What all these records show is that, while we had a relationship with honey bees when we were hunter-gatherers, we took that relationship a major step further just about the time we decided to stay in one place. However, the most fascinating thing to consider is this: there is a distinct possibility that the choice to enter into this relationship may not just have been one way.

The author Michael Pollan has argued that maize/corn 'used' humans to spread itself from its place of origin in Central America. It was capable of living in a range of climates and soils all over the planet. All it needed was a bit of help to get around. And it succeeded by being so very useful to us.*

As it turns out, much the same thing could be said about honey bees, certainly in how we have taken them around the world, and perhaps in some even more direct ways as well. In fact, they may have selected us as much as we selected them. It is quite possible that honey bees found a competitive advantage in choosing nest sites near, and even attached to, human habitations, since of course the hurly-burly of activity, and the presence of those other animal adapters to humans, the dogs, may have kept away a wide range of animal predators of the bees. This is certainly still the case in rural Southeast Asia. If you want to find colonies of the Eastern honey bee (*Apis cerana*), the eaves and nooks and crannies of huts is the best place to search.

And when you look at the clay pots that were being used as beehives in Ancient Egypt, it's not hard to believe that honey bees may long ago have shown us how we could keep them, instead of having to raid their nests up in the trees. We know now that swarms (the way honey bees procreate naturally through the spread of colonies) are very good at searching out cavities of just the right sort of dimensions to successfully house themselves, including sufficient space to accumulate ample honey stores. So it's easy to visualise a swarm settling in an empty and perhaps discarded clay pot. All it would then take is for some enterprising person to move the pot up against a wall, and maybe stack a few more around and on top of it as well. The result would be what we now call an *apiary*.

The good news for us humans would have been a lot less danger getting some honey (except, of course, for the stings). The benefit for the honey bees would not only have been lots of nest sites, but a lot less chance of having their colony destroyed. Our ancestors would have soon learned that if they were careful, and only took out a small portion of honey (rather than the brood and maybe with it the queen), the colony would survive, live on for another year, and produce a few swarms as well.

Storing your fat in your nest

The species we are concerned with in this book is *Apis mellifera*, the Western honey bee. While there is always debate about the total number, the *Apis* genus has at least six other members. The Eastern honey bee mentioned a couple of paragraphs ago is the only other species that is successfully kept in hives, while *Apis dorsata*, the giant honey bee, is the species that is still visited by honey hunters.

Given that all but one of these species have their natural ranges in Asia, the suggestion is that this is the original centre of development of the genus. And what a development it was. These honey bees, along with bumblebees, hundreds of species of wasps, and thousands more of ants, worked out a very different way of living in the world — they became social. Other bee species have remained solitary, meaning that every female has to create a nest, lay eggs, and leave some food behind for when the eggs hatch. To put it bluntly, the 'house' they make isn't a home.

The social species do it very differently. They live together in a colony, and not all members are the same. In the case of the *Apis* species, there are lots of worker bees, which are females that (at least normally) don't lay eggs. This job is carried out by a queen, which mates once in her life with a series of drones (the only male bees), keeps all the sperm from those matings in a special sac called a *spermatheca*, and portions it out internally to fertilise eggs right through her entire life, which can often last several years.*

It sounds like chaos, and it can very occasionally be so if a queen dies or flies away with a swarm, and a new one isn't raised, because it's impossible for worker bees to ever mate with drones and lay fertilised eggs. But what normally keeps everything in order is a chemical the queen produces from glands in her head just behind her mandible, those pinching-like mouth parts on bees. This *queen pheromone* is part birth control (it keeps worker bees from developing their ovaries, and workers from rearing new queens), and part societal glue (it's how bees know where they live and are able to identify intruders).

The other wonderful attribute of honey bees is of course the food they make. For them, it's the other vital part of being 'social'. They don't have to carry fat around with them like we do, and go through a complex process of metabolism to create the energy needed to survive. They have instead worked out a way to store their energy all around them in their nest.

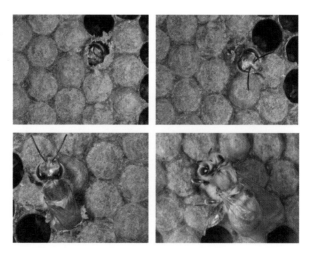

The birth of a worker bee, as it chews its way out of its brood cell by eating the capping. The bee will spend the first three weeks of its life on a variety of colony duties, and the last three weeks flying around the countryside foraging for nectar and pollen.

Lastly, honey bees alone among the insects have worked out a way to communicate visually the location of the best available food sources, using the famous *bee dance*, as well as a built-in time clock, and even dialects, all originally deciphered by the scientist Karl von Frisch. Von Frisch won a Nobel Prize for his efforts in 1973, but the distinctive waggle made by returning foraging bees, which appeared to convey such information as the direction and distance of nectar-bearing flowers, was disputed for years. It was only in 2005, when scientists used harmonic radar to track bees in real time, that this unique ability was confirmed once and for all.*

Apis mellifera is the true master of this whole process. They have lived in cold-temperate climates for at least the last 10–12 million years, and in order to cope with long, harsh winters they have developed the ability to collect and store many kilograms of honey; so many, in fact, that there is usually enough for them to make it through to the spring, as well as provide a goodly amount for us.

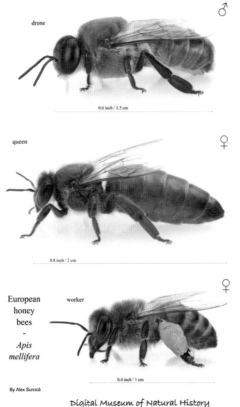

drone ♂

0.6 inch / 1.5 cm

queen ♀

0.8 inch / 2 cm

European honey bees

-

Apis mellifera

By Alex Surcică

worker ♀

0.4 inch / 1 cm

Digital Museum of Natural History

The three honey bee castes: drone, queen and worker bee. Drones are the only male honey bees, and as their name suggests they carry out no duties in the colony apart from waiting for the off-chance to mate with a virgin queen high in the air. Any drone lucky enough to fulfil his destiny dies instantly when the mating takes place.

It is this superior honey gathering, this never producing just enough to survive, that has attracted people to keep honey bee colonies in their tens, and then hundreds, and finally thousands. They are worthwhile enough creatures to have been taken from their original range in Central Europe and sub-Saharan Africa all around the world. Michael Pollan used maize as his example, but he could just as easily have chosen honey bees.

None of the other *Apis* species have ever had such a successful relationship with us. And the Western honey bee has adapted so well to so many climates and flowering plants that they are now present in every continent save Antarctica, and from just below the Arctic Circle to the deepest tropical jungles.

To put it mildly, honey bees and humans have become very, very close. So close, in fact, that if we observe them very thoroughly they have a lot to teach us about making our way in the world.

The truly sustainable 'bi-vore'

Honey bees are remarkable creatures for a number of reasons. But a point that is often forgotten is that they have managed to successfully adapt to a wide range of climates and environmental conditions without needing to kill other animals for food, or even chew on plants. And when they find suitable enclosed shelter from the elements, either naturally, or in something constructed by humans, they also create the additional structures in which to live, raise their young, and store their food supplies, all from a material (*beeswax*) that they produce from their own special glands.

To coin a phrase, honey bees are 'bi-vores', because they make their living entirely by collecting nectar (which is their source of carbohydrate, and which they convert to honey as well as to beeswax) and pollen (which provides them with proteins and minerals, and is used to grow out their larval brood). No other food sources are involved.

And of course plants create those flowers, and produce the nectar and pollen voluntarily, as their means of reproduction through the transferring of genetic material (the strictest definition of the word 'sex'). When all is said and done, plants and honey bees have an almost perfect, mutually beneficial relationship.

The term 'sustainability' is bandied about a lot these days, to the point where you sometimes have to wonder if it hasn't lost its true meaning. That's particularly true when even big companies in industries like mining and oil jump on the sustainability bandwagon. Sustainability in its purest sense is a biological term used to describe well-functioning ecosystems. In such systems 'waste equals food', and the supply of nutrients is recycled between all the plants and animals in such a way that no further inputs, apart from water and sunlight, are needed for the system to carry on indefinitely.

Mankind, especially since the time of the Industrial Revolution, has of course followed a much different path, namely creating fantastic amounts of waste and pollution to produce things that we don't (and often can't) use again. Ecosystems survive and are sustainable because they circulate and re-use energy and materials. Modern industry is unsustainable, because it continues to rely mostly on the one-way street of resource extraction and depletion.

Honey bees, on the other hand, have taken the idea of sustainability to a whole new level. Not only do they not do anything to degrade the ecosystem around them, they add a positive benefit that is essential for many of the plants in that system to survive from one generation to the next. To use the phrase currently fashionable in industrial design, bees don't just recycle, they *up-cycle*, with less truly becoming more.*

Cooking with bees

We humans tend to think we are a special species when it comes to how we handle our food, since we most often transform it in one way or another to make it more digestible and keep it from spoiling. As Michael Pollan says, it's a set of processes we often lump together under the general term 'cooking'. And as anyone who has ever made yogurt, cheese or sauerkraut will tell you, it doesn't necessarily always mean roasting things in the oven or even boiling them on top of the stove.*

However, if you accept that definition, it turns out we're not the only ones who cook. Honey bees transform the raw materials they collect from flowers as well. They may not be cordon bleu chefs, but they're masters at fitting the most amount of nutrient into the least amount of space, and doing things to it to make sure it doesn't

37

spoil. We humans aren't the only animals who are able to preserve food so that we can eat it later on. Honey bees even change nectar and pollen to make it easier to digest, which of course is another reason our ancestors originally learned how to transform the grains, roots and meat we consume.

Nectar as it is produced by plants and secreted in the nectaries of flowers is almost entirely sucrose, a *disaccharide*, meaning that it has two (*di-*) sugar molecules held together by a chemical bond. There are a few other bits and pieces, including small amounts of various proteins, minerals, some pigments, and of course some aromatic substances that give it both smell and taste. Finally, of course, there is also a substantial amount of moisture in the nectar, but this varies considerably depending on the plant itself and the humidity in the atmosphere. It can't be too dilute, however, because somewhat surprisingly a honey bee's ability to detect sweetness (the amount of sugar in a solution) isn't that much better than our own.

Foraging bees (worker honey bees generally in the last half of their adult life) gather the nectar from flowers, sucking it down using a part of their anatomy (the *proboscis*) that some have likened to an elephant's trunk. In this case, however, it's a trunk that can be split into four sections, as well as be tucked below the head when not in use. Foragers are very adept at collecting this nectar, even when the flower itself may have long, tube-shaped petals protecting the nectaries. There are some plant species that make it pretty tough, however, including lucerne (also known as alfalfa) which has the nasty habit of springing a sort of trap-door when it is first visited, giving the bee a thump on the head. Honey bees are excellent learners, however, and either work out how to approach these sorts of flowers from the side, or avoid them entirely.

Honey bees are also *species constant*, meaning that they generally only visit flowers of the same species on any given foraging trip. This helps a bit in giving the honey they eventually produce from the nectar a consistency of taste and flavour, which is nice for us humans. More importantly, it greatly helps the plants themselves, since the transfer of pollen that clings to the bees goes to other flowers of the same species. It is an ability — along with the bee dance identifying the location of crops in flower — that other pollinating insects just don't have.

The nectar itself is held inside the bee in a sac just in front of the bee's stomach. The sac can expand greatly in size, allowing the bee to bring back large amounts of nectar, and the outside plates covering the bee (it's only 'skeleton') can also slide in and out, accommodating the extra girth. The contents of a very full honey sac can reach 70 milligrams, or 85% of the tare weight of the bee, although the average load of nectar during a honey flow is about 40 milligrams. There is also an amazing valve called the *proventriculus*, which separates the honey sac from the stomach, and has the ability to regulate the passage of pollen to be digested as food while still allowing nectar to be retained for transport back to the colony.

When the foraging bee returns to the colony, that's when the transformation process (the 'cooking') begins. To get the most amount of energy into those little hexagonal cells that make up the comb, once the foraging bee has passed over her sacful of nectar to waiting processing bees (younger workers, or those not foraging for whatever reason), they have to evaporate off a lot of excess moisture. They do this by turning the colony into a remarkably efficient dehumidifier.

Each processor pumps a bit of nectar out of her honey sac, and suspends it as a flat drop on the underside of her proboscis. In so doing, a large surface area of the liquid (at least compared with its tiny volume) is exposed to the air. Other bees are busy fanning air around the colony, and heating it to about 34° Celsius. This works best at night, when the temperature of the air outside the colony is lower, and therefore can't hold as much moisture (the reason dew forms on the ground on a cool night). Fanning this air into the colony and heating it makes it able to take on more moisture again, and it acts almost like a sponge, pulling moisture out of the suspended droplets of nectar. This process is repeated rapidly for 15–20 minutes, and as a result the contents of the honey sac loses approximately half of its water. The moisture content is now between 30% and 50%.

The second phase of honey ripening then follows. The bees deposit the half-ripened honey in small droplets on the cell walls,

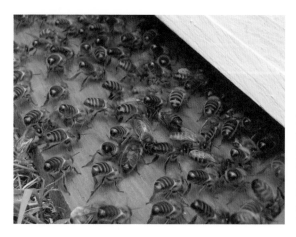

Dehumidifiers, chemical engineers, packaging experts: honey bees have been successfully transforming their food for over 10 million years.

or in a thin film on the cell floor and various other hive surfaces. As a rule, a quarter to a third of the cell is filled. However, during a strong flow, or if there is a lack of space, half to three-quarters of each cell is filled straight away. Normally when the honey is nearly ripe, the bees move it again, and the cells are filled to three-quarters of their capacity.

Only when the honey is fully ripe (that is, is less than 20% moisture), do the bees fill the cells completely and seal them with an airtight wax capping. Since the honey is now super-saturated, that capping is very important, because it will keep the honey in the cell from re-absorbing moisture. It's just like putting a lid on a jar.

If the moisture rises above 20%, the spores of sugar-tolerant yeasts will be able to hatch, starting off the fermentation process. Humans might get a kick out of the alcohol that is produced, but for bees it's toxic, and so they go to great lengths to preserve this essential stored nutrient.

Getting a sugar solution significantly below what is the equilibrium point of 64% is quite an accomplishment for anyone, and not just honey bees. But something just as amazing takes place at the same time — a bit of chemistry. During her collection journey, the foraging bee has already added some special substances from glands in her head, the same glands that earlier in her life she had used to secrete royal jelly for feeding to larvae and the queen. The first of these is called *invertase*, and it really starts to make things happen as the nectar is ripened into honey in the hive. More invertase is added by processing bees and, with the help of the warmth from air being fanned about inside the colony, a reaction begins to takes place. The invertase breaks apart the bonds holding the two sugar molecules (the disaccharide) together in the sucrose-rich nectar, converting almost all of it into the *mono-saccharides* fructose and glucose. Everyone is probably familiar with glucose, since these days it's the high-energy ingredient in most sports drinks. Fructose is also now quite common, because syrup obtained from maize that contains high levels of the sugar is used as the sweetener in fizzy drinks.

Inverting the nectar, and then storing it as an extremely dense liquid makes a lot of sense from the bees' point of view. What they have done in effect is pre-digest the sugar, so that when it is ingested it provides them with an instant source of energy. The same holds true for us humans. When we eat sucrose, before our cells can use the carbohydrate to create energy we first need to process it in our stomach and break apart those bonds. We in fact have to use energy to produce energy. When we eat honey, on the other hand, the bees have already done that work for us. Research has even shown that we can absorb these single molecules directly through the mucous membranes in our mouth, short-circuiting the stomach route entirely.

But if all that weren't enough, bees also add another enzyme to the nectar during the ripening process, an enzyme that is very important in giving honey at least part of its antibacterial activity. An enzyme called *glucose oxidase* also comes from those multi-purpose head glands, and it changes some of the glucose into a substance that becomes *gluconic acid*. This acidity, which we mentioned in the previous chapter ('if honey wasn't so sweet it would taste sour'), helps protect the nectar from fermenting during the ripening process while it is still fairly high in moisture.

But that's not all glucose oxidase does. This is also the enzyme that produces hydrogen peroxide in honey, the antimicrobial substance that Peter Molan and Kerry Simpson had to knock out when they were doing those first tests on New Zealand honey. While the glucose oxidase the bees add helps prevent fermentation during ripening, what's really great is that, so long as the honey hasn't been over-heated during extraction and packing, it remains present in the final product, and can start producing hydrogen peroxide again if and when the honey becomes diluted. The action of the enzyme then increases dramatically (from 2500 to 50,000 times), providing a slow-release of hydrogen peroxide that produces the antibacterial effect.*

The bakery in the hive

When it comes to turning nectar into honey, the bee colony is nothing short of a food-processing factory. To complete the picture, however, we also need to spend a couple of paragraphs describing two more transformations they manage to achieve.

The first has to do with pollen, the other half of the bees' bi-vore food equation. A honey bee colony reaches a maximum population of about 60,000 individual bees at the height of the summer honey flows, and, since worker bees only live for about six weeks, to achieve that population growth there's a major need for protein, vitamins and minerals to feed all those hungry larval mouths, as well as to keep up the royal jelly intake so that the queen is able to lay 1500 to 2000 eggs per day.

Thankfully for the world at large, and our own enthusiasm for fruits and vegetables, honey bees are able to gather the raw materials for all that brood and queen food from the pollen produced by thousands of species of flowering plants. Some of that pollen is collected inadvertently as honey bees gather nectar, since pollen grains are fairly sticky, and the bee quite fortuitously is covered with lots of trap-like branched hairs that look a bit like tiny Christmas trees.

Much more, however, is collected by bees very purposely, either on the same trip as they gather nectar, or sometimes on trips made just for pollen alone. The bees will even grab the anthers (the part of the flower that produces the pollen) with their mandibles, and scrabble around in an effort to get as much pollen on themselves as possible.

Honey bees also have some great anatomical devices that let them collect all those pollen grains into neat packages to more easily carry them back home. As it turns out, humans aren't the only ones who use combs and brushes on their often unruly hair. Bees have the same sorts of things built into their legs, and if you watch them closely as they fly from flower to flower, you can see them pause in mid-air and go through a set of acrobatic contortions. They comb themselves with their front two sets of legs, then, using brushes on their back legs, combine the pollen grains together with a bit of nectar and press them around a long single hair, the well-known (but erroneously named) pollen 'basket'.

It's at this stage that *bee pollen* becomes recognisable to us, as brightly-coloured pellets, each containing millions of individual grains of pollen. The weight of pellets can sometimes be as much as 30 milligrams. At two pellets per loaded bee, that's not as heavy as a full honey sac of nectar, but carrying it is still quite an accomplishment, especially when you consider that during good weather, over 50,000 such loads are brought into the colony in a day. And the total yearly requirement of a honey bee colony can be as much as 30 kilograms.

The foraging bees carry the pellets back home, and then literally head-butt the pellets into wax cells in the comb, along with the same enzymes used with nectar to inhibit germination and spoilage. Once the cell is filled (and this will take a series of loads), a thin layer of honey is put over the pollen, and here's where another little bit of food processing and preservation takes place. In the comb the stored pollen undergoes partial anaerobic fermentation, preserving the pollen in a form known as *bee bread*. The fermentation produces lactic acid in the pollen, increasing both acidity and water-soluble

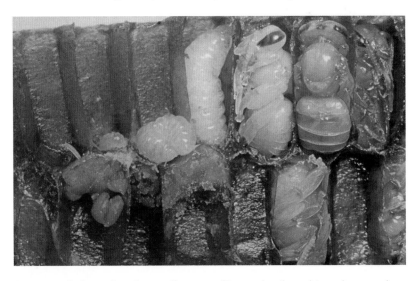

An unusual photo that shows all stages of honey bee brood (egg, larva and pupa) as well as pollen pellets that foraging bees have deposited in cells ready to be consumed by nurse bees.

protein. Anyone brave enough to smell the air that bees circulate out the front entrance of their hive at the end of a good foraging day will know the distinctive smell associated with this fermentation. Picking up on the bee bread analogy, it's the honey bee version of the fragrance that wafts from a bakery.

An insect that self-medicates

Honey bees obviously have things very well worked out when it comes to the foods they need to survive. They are so efficient, in fact, that it can come as a surprise to learn they forage for one extra plant material they have determined is essential for their survival, something that they don't eat at all.

In every colony a small number of foraging bees make trips to trees and shrubs, hunting for resin that the plants either use to protect new and tender leaves (the sticky capsule covering poplar buds is a good example), or that the plants secrete when there has been some damage to the bark covering of their woody structures (a response that might be compared to our body producing a scab).

What these resins are part of, in fact, is the immune systems of these trees and shrubs. They contain compounds that aren't just highly antibacterial; they have an ability to kill fungi and viruses as well.

Bees go out of their way to collect these resins, no matter where in the world they happen to live, and bring them back to the colony

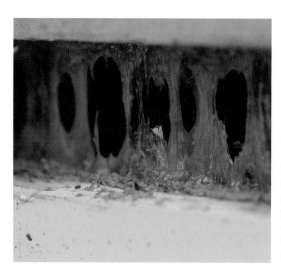

Sticky propolis when two bee boxes are prised apart. Propolis is formed from resins collected by bees, not just to seal holes and entomb intruders, but as a means of self-medication as well.

where they combine them with their own beeswax. They use the resulting material as a kind of plaster, filling gaps, closing up holes, and even covering over dead intruders like bumblebees or mice that the bees are unable to tear apart and remove. It's the reason beekeepers use a special lever (the *hive tool*) to work their way through beehives. The resin and wax mixtures sticks all the hive parts together like glue. This substance is called *propolis*, thanks to beekeepers in ancient Greece who observed that bees used it to close down and protect hive entrances (*pro* = in front, or in defence of; *polis* = the city).

We now know that propolis is one of the most complex and potent biological substances ever studied. Over 350 different compounds have been identified, and it has been shown to not only be antimicrobial, but anti-inflammatory as well. Propolis is one of the strongest natural antioxidants, and in the laboratory it has even been shown to be effective in inhibiting the growth of a wide range of cancer cells.

The question, though, is why do the bees go to the trouble of collecting this single material in addition to the nectar and pollen that satisfies all the rest of their needs? It has always been assumed that propolis had a purpose in addition to stopping up gaps, since it has been shown to kill a range of pathogens that cause diseases specific to honey bees. However, only recently have scientists been able to design experiments that proved for the first time that honey bees really do use propolis to *self-medicate.**

Bees, booze and medicine

The realisation that honey bees may not just be excellent food processors, but use the plants around them as a kind of pharmacy as well, brings us around quite nicely to our own species' long and involved history using bee products as medicine.

And returning to the theme of our relationship with the bees, it's not outside the realm of possibility that ancient man (and woman) may even have got the idea of using honey for therapeutic purposes from the bees themselves. Spoiled food was (and still is) a huge problem, and yet here was a food product that in the beehive stayed perfectly fine. Even when harvested it didn't require any cooking or salting or pickling. It had a special power that many other foods just couldn't match, a power our ancestors appear to have thought was magical.

In fact, the worst that can be said for honey is that if it sits around long enough in a wet climate without being covered it can start to develop a tangy fizz, and that most definitely helped our forbears to develop a taste for the tipple. The famous anthropologist Claude Lévi-Strauss has even argued that honey-based alcohol was a crucial element in the move from a hunter-gatherer nomadic lifestyle to a more sedentary existence with permanent settlements. Alcoholic honey drinks most probably also pre-dated the invention of bread, that other major food transformation involving yeast.*

We can have little idea about the full range of ways our pre-historic ancestors used honey; only that they went to great efforts and sometimes great risk to obtain it. It was, after all, the most intensely sweet thing available, and remained so until the advent of sugar production from cane sugar in the 1700s.

What we do know for sure, however, is that once records began being kept, honey most definitely had what archaeologists call *magico-religious significance* for many ancient civilisations. Honey is mentioned repeatedly in the sacred books of most religious traditions, including Hinduism ('Let one take honey to beautify his appearance, develop his brain faculty, and strengthen his body' — *Rig Veda* 1:90:6–8); Buddhism (the Festival of Madhu Purnima celebrates the Buddha receiving honeycomb from a monkey during his retreat to the wilderness seeking to create peace amongst his disciples); Judaism ('Eat thou honey because it is good' — *Proverbs* 24:13); Islam ('From inside the dwellings of bees comes a drink of many colours, containing healing for mankind' — *Koran* 16:69); and Christianity (the first foods Christ was given after his resurrection were honeycomb and fish — *Luke* 24:42–43).

As well, beginning with the very earliest written records, honey is given prominence as a medicine. In fact, a clay tablet found in the Tigris-Euphrates valley in Mesopotamia, and dating from around 2100 BC, provides arguably the world's first prescriptions, including a recipe for wound treatment using honey.

In Ancient Egypt, honey was so important that, beginning in the First Dynasty (3200 BC), the bee was used as the sign of the king of Lower Egypt, and was displayed in hieroglyphs in temples. Priests used honey in religious rites, and in the Ebers Papyrus (scrolls dating from 1550 BC), honey is listed as an ingredient in no less than 140 different medical preparations, including wound dressings following surgery (including circumcision), a treatment for hair loss due to fungal infections, salves for abscesses, and even a suppository (presumably to treat haemorrhoids).

The Smith Papyrus, a remarkable scroll from about the same time, is the oldest known medical text describing surgery and treatments for trauma. It even presents case studies, just like medical journals do today. One such case describes how honey was used to treat a deep wound extending to the bone that included stitches. The papyrus also describes the use of bandages woven from linen, which were soaked in honey and frankincense, and offers a gargle using the same ingredients (along with aniseed) as a mouthwash to treat canker sores.

Clearly honey was an important part of the Egyptian way of life. As time went on, the product became more common place, and its use wasn't confined just to royalty and the upper classes. In fact, beekeeping became so well developed that eventually hives were taken up the Nile on rafts every October, and slowly brought back down as the bees took advantage of the progression of flowering crops, reaching Cairo in February, where the accumulated production was offered for sale. The Egyptians were thus not only some of the first beekeepers, but the first to practise migratory beekeeping as well.

Honey, beeswax and propolis were also used in the preparation of the dead, not just in the famous Egyptian mummies, but also in the preserving of many other famous figures from antiquity. For instance, it is said that the body of Alexander the Great was brought back from Babylon in a coffin filled with honey, and the King of ancient Sparta, King Herod, and Nero's wife were embalmed with honey as well.

Mellarius, fetch me a (honey)comb

The Ancient Greeks were great observers and writers, giving us some of the first investigations concerning the natural world. The greatest Greek philosopher of them all, and some might say the world's first scientist, was Aristotle, and he spent considerable time observing honey bees, trying to work out where honey came from, including the fact that bees collect nectar from flowers, take it back to the colony in their honey sac, regurgitate it into cells, and convert it from a thin liquid resembling water to a thick substance that can be recognised by its taste. What he got wrong, strangely, was the idea that the nectar itself wasn't produced by plants. He thought it was deposited in flowers from the atmosphere.

As you can imagine, the Greek physician Hippocrates also had a few things to say about honey, including that it 'cleans sores and ulcers, softens hard ulcers of the lips, heals carbuncles and running sores'. He prescribed honey and vinegar (which he called 'Oxymel') as a topical application to reduce pain, and honey and water ('Hydromel') to treat thirst associated with fever.

Honey really came into its own as a medicine, however, during the Roman Empire. It was one of the most useful substances listed in the Roman pharmacopoeia, where it was prescribed both on its own and together with a range of other substances. The physician Celsus used honey as a cure for diarrhoea, and the writer Pliny the Elder (AD 23–79) recommended that honey be used for a range of ailments, including respiratory infections, quinsy (abscesses associated with tonsillitis), and even inflammation caused by snake bites. He also noted that, while some honeys may not have an appealing taste, they often would make a good topical treatment for bruises and the like.

Discordes, a Greek physician writing during the height of the Roman Empire, prescribed honey for a number of conditions, including many that the product is still used for today. They included sores, leg ulcers, and throat, tonsil and eye infections. Discordes also presaged what modern scientific investigation has shown us, namely that not all honeys have the same level of curative properties.

Beekeeping was also very popular during the Roman Empire, and landowners often had a special slave called a *mellarius* to tend their hives and collect honey. For the first time, considerable writing took place regarding beekeeping practices, and something from that time still exists in apiculture today. Around the world, the most popular variety of honey bee is the 'Italian' (*Apis mellifera ligustica*), which originated in the Iberian Peninsula, and was surely used in Roman times.*

Trading honey for silk, and the town that put out a fire with mead

Honey has always been precious in Chinese civilisation. But while in ancient times it was greatly revered, it was not easy to come by because the one species of indigenous honey bee (*Apis cerana*) that beekeepers could coax into living in hives didn't produce large quantities of honey, and often wouldn't stay put. Robbing honey from the giant colonies of *Apis dorsata*, on the other hand, was a job only for the very brave. Numerous accounts exist from various dynasties of such escapades, including trying to access a wild nest by being lowered over the side of a cliff in a chair.

The difficulty in collecting and producing honey is perhaps the reason that, in the first century, the product was recorded as one of the main imports into the kingdom from the West, and was traded for silk. It also helps explain why honey has always been highly prized as a medicine in Chinese and other East Asian cultures, rather than as simply a food.

The medicinal uses of bee products are described in the *Divine Farmer's Materia Medica* (*Shennong Bencao Jing*). The book's

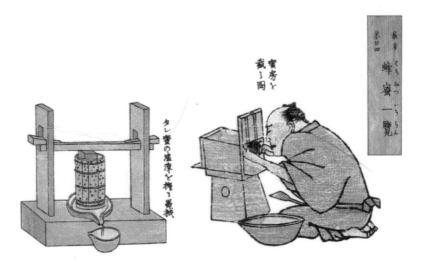

Traditional hive beekeeping in Asia involved the keeping of *Apis cerana*, as this woodblock from Japan charmingly depicts.

origin has been attributed to the Chinese sovereign Shennong, who was said to have lived around 2800 BC. However, researchers hypothesise that it is in fact a compilation of oral traditions, and was written between about 300 BC and AD 200. Honey is indicated in a number of cases, and acts according to the principles of the Earth element. It is said to boost the *qi*, or life force, relieve pain and harmonise hundreds of medicinals.*

Honey was also prominent in the Ayurvedic medicine first developed in ancient India. As early as 1400 BC, the surgeon Susrata identified eight different types of honey produced by different bee species, and from different plant sources. To each variety he ascribed different medical properties, including relieving fever, treating coughs, and alleviating skin diseases. The *Ashtanga Hridaya*, from about the 7th century AD, recommended honey for the cleaning and covering of wounds, as well as for a range of infections, internal and external.

In the Americas before the time of Columbus, honey was also an important commodity, even though there were no *Apis* species indigenous to the New World. Instead, a separate group of social bees had evolved there that made nests and produced at least small amounts of honey. The group is now commonly called the *stingless bees*. Despite the name, however, they are not without defences. Some species scare predators by getting into their hair, while others squirt a repelling scent. Another tactic involves crawling deep within the poor unfortunate's ear canal and then buzzing. As rural children in South America will tell you even today, once you experience it you will remember forever after to seal up your ears with whatever comes to hand (fingers included).

The Mayans greatly prized honey and beeswax, and the ubiquitous yeasts provided them with inebriating results when water was added to honey and left to stand for a while. They even had two different honey festivals in their famous calendar, one in October/December to hopefully improve the coming crop, and the other in January/February to drink honey wine.

The Aztecs also utilised the same sort of honey, and their most important medicinal tonic consisted of cacao bean powder, vanilla,

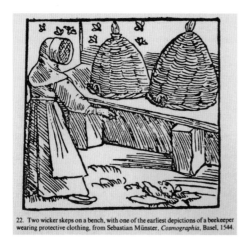

22. Two wicker skeps on a bench, with one of the earliest depictions of a beekeeper wearing protective clothing, from Sebastian Münster, *Cosmographia*, Basel, 1544.

Beekeeping was widespread in Europe during the Middle Ages, and honey was the only real sweetener until the advent of sugar cane plantations in the Caribbean in the 1700s.

pepper and honey. Cortés reported that honey and beeswax were on sale in the Aztec markets.

Species of stingless bees can also be found in Africa, Asia and Australia. On that last continent, Aboriginal tribes consider honey to be the supreme delicacy, and they also eat bee larvae and pupae, both of which have high protein content.*

There are very few references to the therapeutic uses of the honey during the Dark Ages, but that's hardly surprising. Medical developments, like most intellectual enquiry, were subjugated to the temporal authority of the Catholic Church. As Eva Crane, the world's foremost authority on honey, has said, 'It was the Arabs, and later the Moors, who built the shining bridge which spans the Dark Ages; they passed on to the rest of Europe the learning of Ancient Greece, including what was known about bees and honey.'* Arab physicians routinely prescribed honey, including for stomach complaints, and to treat tonsillitis.

That is not to say, of course, that beekeeping didn't carry on in Europe, and that honey wasn't an important product. Quite the contrary. The Church itself had a strong demand for beeswax for candles. And while historians in the past have claimed that very little honey was consumed by the general population, a recent re-evaluation of the evidence suggests that may not have been the case.* Many farms would have had their own beehives, while in some parts of England honey was used to pay rent.

And as anyone who has read *Beowulf* will know, mead made from honey was a well known and very much enjoyed drink. It was so plentiful in some parts that in 1015, in the German city of Meissen, mead (or at least honey beer) was used to put out a fire because the townspeople had more of it to hand than they did water.* That may sound preposterous until you realise that fermented beverages with low alcoholic content were the drink of choice in the Middle Ages for adults and even children, since drinking water often led to dysentery and even worse. Beer was even regarded as a major source of sustenance. In the making of many of these brewed drinks, honey was the only real sugary substance in northern Europe until cane sugar became readily available following the development of plantations in the Caribbean.*

With the advent of the Enlightenment, a book appeared in England on the subject of beekeeping that is still regarded as a classic. *The Feminine Monarchie*, written by the Reverend Charles Butler in the early 1600s, not only propounded the startling theory that the honey bee colony was headed up by a queen, rather than by a king; it also went into great detail about the medical uses of honey, including its effectiveness as a cough medicine and treatment for sore throats.

The great beekeeping revolution

In the middle of the nineteenth century a great revolution occurred in beekeeping. It started in America, and quickly travelled around the globe. While the Western world now had cane sugar well and truly at its disposal, honey production also increased, especially as beekeeping became readily established in the New World. It also became truly commercial, with the advent of the moveable frame hive, popularised (if not perhaps actually invented) by the Reverend L. L. Langstroth.*

At the time, Langstroth was the principal at a school for young ladies in Philadelphia, and had taken up beekeeping as a hobby to distract himself during bouts of depression. In the autumn of 1851, he made his crucial discovery. If the wooden frames holding combs of beeswax, as well as all the other internal dimensions of a hive, were kept to the same width as the spacing that wild colonies made between their combs, bees could be kept in hives that could be easily taken apart and put back together again. He called the gap *bee space*, a distance of precisely 3/8 inch, or 9.5 millimetres. He recorded in his diary on that day the realisation of what was in fact an 'almost self-evident idea ... seeing by intuition, as it were, the end from the beginning, I could scarcely refrain from shouting out my "Eureka!" in the open streets'.

For the first time since our ancestors first managed to coax a swarm of bees to live inside a man-made object at least four thousand years ago, beekeepers could go into the hive, check its condition and food stores, try to control its diseases, and most importantly, remove the surplus honey crop, all without damaging (often fatally) the colony itself.

Through systematic queen-rearing and the making of splits, hive numbers could purposely be doubled or even trebled in the spring period leading up to the honey flow. Skeps, the up-turned straw baskets that had become a symbol of bees and beekeeping, especially in Europe, would soon become a thing of the past. The modern age of beekeeping, as we still pretty much know it today, had begun.

So far as the medical use of products from those hives was concerned, however, very little was commented on during this period. Honey was in common use, both in the home and by medical

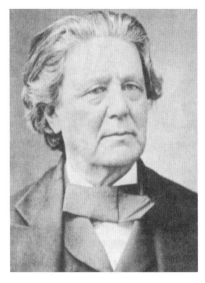

Lorenzo Lorraine Langstroth, the clergyman and school principal from Philadelphia whose invention of the moveable frame hive started a world-wide revolution in beekeeping.

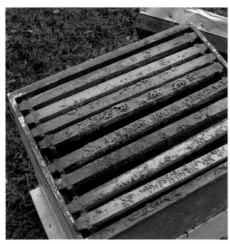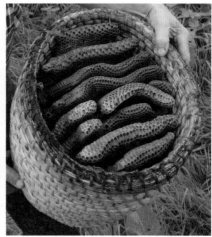

The 'bee space' honey bees leave in natural comb (in this case in a straw skep), gave Langstroth the idea of providing the same spacing for combs in wooden frames. Provided the same bee space was maintained throughout all parts of the hive, bees wouldn't fill the gaps with comb, and the beekeeper could easily manipulate the hive, adding extra boxes for increased honey production.

practitioners, particularly in the treatment of wounds and burns. For instance, in New Zealand it was part of standard woundcare practice in hospitals prior to World War II.* And honey itself was shown to be antibacterial as far back as 1892, only a decade or so after Koch used his postulates to prove bacteria could cause disease.*

What changed everything, however, at least in the West, was the advent of antibiotics. The 'wonder drugs' of the age were used to treat all sorts of diseases and conditions, and saved countless lives. Pharmaceutical companies and the medical establishment seemed so victorious that in 1969 the US Surgeon General could confidently state, 'The time has come to close the book on infectious disease.'* Honey, on the other hand, seemed to have been relegated to something you put on toast. In the East there was no problem understanding that food could also be medicine. But in the West, while there were more honey bees in more places than there had ever been, honey was now regarded as only a food. And given that sugar production worldwide had now displaced honey by a factor of 100 to 1, it was verging on being a niche item at that.* So far as honey's use in medicine was concerned, it was put in the category of an interesting historical curiosity.

As we know now, however, the war we have with bacteria is far from over. They have been around a lot longer than we have (several billion years longer, in fact), make up much more of the biological world, and are extremely adept at overcoming all sorts of difficulties. If you can work out how to live at the bottom of the ocean in steam vents at temperatures of over 100° Celsius, man-made chemicals designed to kill you aren't likely to pose too much of a threat long-term.*

And so it was towards the end of the twentieth century that the advent of antibiotic-resistant bacteria, especially ones associated with wounds and sores that just wouldn't heal, made some medical soldiers at the frontlines (otherwise known as nurses) begin to think again. They could remember stories about the use of honey in hospitals, and a few had recently tried it on supposedly hopeless cases, with surprisingly positive results. As well, a professor in New Zealand had discovered a particular variety that seemed to have an amazing ability to kill the very sorts of bacteria that were causing so much woe. It had a peculiar name, and most people had never heard of it. It was manuka. But for some reason, most beekeepers in that country avoided producing it if they possibly could.

Three

GIVING THE
STUFF AWAY

Great Barrier Island is one of the oft-forgotten treasures of New Zealand. As its name suggests, it sits at the far end of the Hauraki Gulf, protecting that world-famous playground for sailing enthusiasts from the storms that generate in the South Pacific Ocean off to the east. It has wonderful bays and coves, a windswept east coast beach, and that special aquamarine colour you see in the water when the sun shines that can't help but make you sigh.

These days it pretty much relies on tourism, with two-thirds of the island in the Conservation Estate. But in the past it was exploited for copper and its kauri, that enormous and slow-growing native tree species whose timber proved exceptional in the building of boats. The Barrier, as locals call it, also had one of the earliest farm settlements in the country, with 40-acre allotments given to ex-soldiers who had served in the New Zealand Wars. Many of the blocks proved too small to be profitable, particularly with the deep clay and thin topsoil, so various other rural activities were also pursued. One of those was beekeeping, and Great Barrier Island had arguably the first commercial beekeeping enterprise in the young country. Several families were involved, and they quickly built up their hive numbers, using that moveable frame system recently popularised by Langstroth in America. They even had their own sawmill on the island, which they used to manufacture both their *frames* (the wooden surrounds that hold the combs) and *supers* (the boxes that hold the frames, so-called because you 'super-impose' one on top of another to increase the size of the hive). They were all made from kauri, a wood that today is as rare as it is prized.

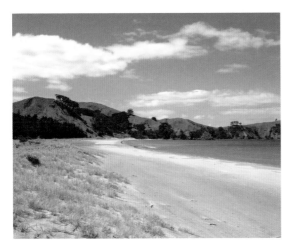

Great Barrier Island, scene of some of the earliest commercial beekeeping in New Zealand, and the source of both manuka honey for the Auckland market, and pohutukawa honey presented to King George V.

Honey production was impressive. In the 1895 season, for instance, the Blackwell family produced 10 tons, with much of it exported to England. Honey was also packed in 2-pound tins and taken to Auckland, eventually being transported on Adam Blackwells launch, *The Rosella*, which became known as the 'honey boat'. Much of the product was sold right at the city's wharf, and it was also carried by a select group of grocery stores.

Great Barrier Island honey was of two sorts. The later crop came from the pohutukawa trees that peppered the coastline, seemingly capable of existing on sheer rock. The big, bright-red flowers that bloom just before Christmas are quintessentially Kiwi, at least in the north half of the North Island, and they produce so much nectar that at times it can literally drip onto the ground. The honey the bees make from those flowers is almost a water-white liquid, or it would be, except for that fact that it granulates very quickly, sometimes while it is still in the comb. The reason is that, after the bees invert it with their special enzyme, it is very high in glucose, and glucose is the sugar in honey that solidifies. If handled properly, however, pohutukawa honey is highly prized. A sample of it, supplied by the Blackwells, was even presented to King George V. And some say in its flavour you can faintly detect the taste of the sea.*

The first crop, on the other hand, came from manuka, a bushy tree that was present throughout the island; in swampland, on clay banks, and as the first real plant that colonised places where the native bush and its kauri had been cleared. While even today manuka (and its close relative kanuka) make up almost half of the vegetation on the island, it was regarded as scrub, and not worth much apart from use as firewood. But at least the bees seemed to like it.*

As a honey, manuka was quite different; it just wouldn't extract easily out of the combs. With pohutukawa (provided it hadn't granulated) or clover, or pretty much any other sort, all you needed to do was trim off the wax the bees had used to cap over the honey-containing cells, then put it into a machine called an *extractor*; basically a really big canister, with a metal frame inside that spun on bearings when you turned an attached handle. Just as happens during the spin cycle in an automatic washing machine, centrifugal force did the rest. With manuka, on the other hand, the job was arduous, to say the least. Combs had to be cut out of the frames, then put into a big double-boiler called a copper, similar to what everyone back then used to wash their clothes in. Once the wax and honey mixture was sufficiently molten, it was ladled into a muslin bag that sat in a contraption resembling a hand cheese-press. The screw was slowly turned on the press, and the honey oozed out the sides.

Thankfully people in Auckland in the early days didn't seem to mind the taste of manuka honey, or 'tea-tree honey' as it was commonly called. It was sold as 'bush blend', often combined with honey from the native rewarewa. But around the time of World War I, the market began to change. There was a lot more honey available in the shops, much of it from clover pastures, especially in the South Island. It was white, and very creamy, and didn't have nearly as strong a taste. Even as early as 1910 it was fetching a market price of 4 pence a pound, while 'bush' sold for half that amount.*

With the advent of World War II, and the mobilisation of much of the male workforce on the Barrier, most of the island's beehives became abandoned. A small but enterprising industry that had once imported special Italian queen bees from America, along with a hand foundation press for making the hexagonal wax sheets (called *foundation*) needed each year to replace the honey comb that was cut out of the frames, had almost ceased to be.

There was a story, though, of someone who decided to collect a crop of honey from what was left, sometime early in the 1950s.

He went through all the effort of taking what full frames he could find off some hives, pressing the manuka honey out of the combs, and putting it into 60-pound tins, the standard container in those days for supply of bulk honey to the Internal Marketing Division, the government agency tasked with finding sales for surplus honey, both within New Zealand and abroad. It is said that he had his crop waiting at the wharf at Tryphena, the only real township on the island, when he received word of the price he would be paid once it arrived at the depot in Auckland; a price so low that it would hardly have covered the cost of the ferry ride. So either in a fit of pique, or as a protest, he dragged the heavy tins to the edge of the pier, and one by one dropped them into the sea.

The story of that deep-sixing of the manuka honey is apocryphal. Knowledge of its truthfulness (or otherwise) seems to have gone to the grave with its teller some years ago. Les Blackwell, the sharp-witted 82-year-old descendant of the Barrier beekeeping clan, swears it never happened. So it can only be regarded as an urban (or more rightly 'rural') legend. Like many such myths, however, it also contains at least a small kernel of truth. And it is certainly telling that, when other longtime New Zealand beekeepers hear the story, they don't necessarily discount it. As Les himself recalls, there was at least one beekeeper on the Barrier who was still trying to make a go of beekeeping following the war, and after being paid 6 pence/1 farthing a pound for his crop by the 'Infernal' Marketing Division, he swore he would never sell his honey to the government again.

It seems almost impossible to believe these days, with manuka honey so sought after all around the world (and beekeeping on Great Barrier Island once again a vibrant industry), but as late as 1990 it was sometimes the case that you literally had to give the stuff away. To explain why, we need to take a journey of discovery, looking back at the history of beekeeping in New Zealand. In doing so we'll discover how honey fell in with the prevailing economic philosophy of the time that affected almost all the country's international trade.

And we'll also see how honey became a test case for a new idea, one that changed the way New Zealanders saw themselves. No longer destined to just be growers and grazers, they found they could market and brand and even retail what they produced — and the world just loved what they made.

A beekeeper called Bumby

Given humans' extraordinarily long relationship with bees and honey, it may come as something of a surprise to realise that no one had ever tasted manuka honey until a little over 170 years ago. The reason is simply that honey bees aren't indigenous to New Zealand, and since they are the creatures that make honey, the substance just didn't exist.

The vast forests and windswept coasts of those three islands that set sail 80 million years ago from the rest of Gondwanaland, in what the English naturalist David Bellamy calls 'Moa's Ark', aren't entirely bee-less, however.* Along with those famous (and now extinct) flightless moa, flowering trees and shrubs not found anywhere else in the world, and many species of birds that get at least some of their food requirements from those flowers' nectar, New Zealand hosts at least 28 different species of native bees, comprising of three genera. The only problem, at least so far as we sweet-loving humans are concerned, is that none of these bees are honey makers. They are all members of that grouping we talked about earlier called 'solitary bees'. They utilise pollen and a bit of nectar, but don't create combs or even live together in colonies. So before anyone could taste honey from New Zealand, that special beneficial relationship between our two species had to once again come into play. People from Europe needed to bring honey bees to the country, just as they were doing all over the rest of the world. And as we'll see shortly, the very first honey those bees produced was most likely manuka.

Not many New Zealanders have heard of Mangungu, let alone know of its importance in the history of the country. Situated on the south bank of the upper reaches of Hokianga Harbour in Northland, these days it is a sleepy settlement, with a pier jutting out amongst the mangroves and what some people claim is the country's oldest pub just down the road.*

In 1827, however, Eruera Maihi Patuone, a Maori chief of the Ngapuhi *iwi* (tribe) took a noble step. He gave permission and protection to English followers of that great reformer and founder of Methodism, John Wesley, in the setting up of a mission station at Mangungu. The Ngapuhi village of Horeke was nearby, and with the help of these locals, in three years a number of buildings were constructed at the mission, including houses, a school, and a carpenter's shop. Gardens and an orchard were planted, and a cemetery was established. Unfortunately, a decade on the main house burnt to the ground in an accidental fire, a not uncommon occurrence in the days when candles and oil lamps were the only source of illumination. But a replacement house was soon built, just in time for the arrival of a new superintendent of missions from Britain, along with his housekeeper, who quite properly also happened to be his sister.

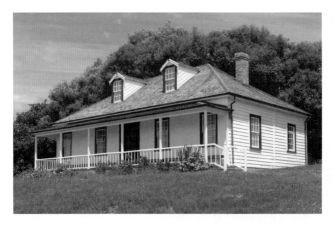

Mangungu Mission House, on the upper reaches of Hokianga Harbour. The first honey ever produced in New Zealand came from hives kept at the mission, a honey that probably had its source in the flowers of nearby stands of manuka scrub. It likely would have been on offer at the house when the Treaty of Waitangi was signed at the grounds on 12 February 1840.

A year later, on 12 February 1840, the mission played host to a great meeting between Ngapuhi chiefs and the representative of the British Crown, Lieutenant Governor William Hobson. It was one of the largest gatherings at the time of Maori and Pakeha (the Maori name for Europeans), and in the end 70 chiefs signed a document that would become known as the Treaty of Waitangi (even though this signing at Mangungu was larger than the more famous one, which had taken place on the opposite coast, in the Bay of Islands, six days before).

Mangungu should therefore rightly hold pride of place for its role in the founding of modern New Zealand. But as it turns out it is also highly significant in our own little story, for a very different reason. When the good ship *James* from Gravesend, England anchored off the mangroves at the mission station in March 1839, that housekeeper who had accompanied her missionary brother brought something very special with her when she disembarked. Her brother loved honey, and the mission church could certainly use some beeswax candles. So amongst the meagre household belongings she managed to take on the voyage, she had included two skeps, those woven straw hives that were common at the time throughout Europe. Inside the skeps was something truly remarkable: two colonies of honey bees that had miraculously survived the six-month journey on a sailing ship all the way from England. The woman herself could hardly have had a better name, at least for the purposes of our tale — she was Mary Bumby, and she was the very first person in New Zealand to ever keep honey bees.

Mary's diary has been lost, and so we have no details about how she managed to look after her charges on that long voyage, or even how the bees took to their new home. We do know what she looked like, however, since her portrait now hangs on the restored mission house at Mangungu. It shows off Mary's bright cheeks, which one

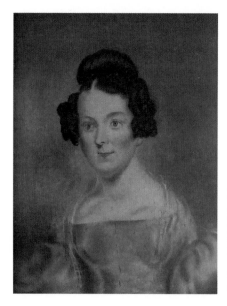

Mary Bumby, New Zealand's first beekeeper. Her bright cheeks gave her the nickname 'The Bonny English Rose', but her brother's love of honey ensured that she brought two skeps of honey bees on an arduous ship's journey all the way from England.

of her contemporaries said entitled her to be called 'The Bonny English Rose'. Mary was also known for her cheerful disposition, and her love of children. A letter written by the daughter of the head of mission many years later, a Mrs Gittos, recalls being taken to see 'the bees from England' soon after the hives' arrival, and sometime later her family received a package from Miss Bumby. In it was a special treat — 'We tried for the first time in our lives real honey in the comb.'

We also know that, as housekeeper, Mary Bumby played host to Governor Hobson that next year at the signing of the Treaty. The hives would have settled in over the winter and collected most of their crop of honey the next season by then, since summer comes very early in Northland. And even today, manuka honey of the very best quality (and highest level of antibacterial activity) comes from the local area, so it is more than likely that this type of honey is what she would have harvested as well. Without a doubt, manuka honey would therefore have been the first honey ever produced in New Zealand. One can only speculate, but given Mary's keenness in sharing her beekeeping bounty, the time of year, and the illustrious visitors present at the station, it's not outside the realm of possibility to think that she may have served manuka honey on the occasion, either in tea or perhaps on bread. Certainly her brother (the Reverend John Bumby) would have approved.

No one knows how long those first beehives remained at Mangungu. John tragically lost his life just four months later, when he and seven others drowned while attempting to cross the Hauraki Gulf. They had been visiting southern mission stations and decided to save time by taking the water route.

By the end of the year, Mary had married Gideon Smales, a young missionary who earlier had been given the sad duty of informing Mary of her brother's death. They were posted to another mission station at Pakanae, had a family, and lived in New Zealand for a further 21 years. Mary died at sea on her way back to England in 1862.*

Bees ahoy!

While Mary Bumby's skeps have become lost in the mists of time, there can be no doubt about what happened to the honey bees they contained, along with a number of other such importations that were made at almost the same time from Australia (where honey bees had been introduced not long before, in 1822).*

To say that this new creature — selected over the centuries to survive the periodic carving out of large portions of its nest by humans keen on its honey stores, and having been miserly enough with its own provisions to withstand an ocean voyage of almost half a year — adapted to the New Zealand environment is something of an understatement. As one observer of the time reported, 'They have increased to such an extent, as to have become wild and fill the forest, so that the bee may be said to be already more established in New Zealand than it is even in England, where it requires much care to preserve it through the winter. Whereas in the mildness of the New Zealand climate, it is quite as much at home in its forest mansions as in its artificial ones.'* Another new immigrant (and the author of New Zealand's first book on beekeeping) was the Reverend William Charles Cotton. He obviously had ample time to watch over his new livestock, since he reported that one colony threw out a total of 26 swarms (the species' natural means of spread) in one year, an almost impossible occurrence back in Britain.*

For the honey bee, New Zealand was an untouched paradise, with plenty of nest sites in the form of holes in trees, no natural predators save for the inquisitive but easily dispelled probings of young boys, and a range of floral sources many of which had evolved to offer enough nectar to feed birds, rather than just insects. This variety of honey bee, the European black (*Apis mellifera mellifera*) became the ubiquitous feral honey bee throughout all of New Zealand for the next 150 years. Many New Zealanders in later generations, who first encountered the bee with a combination of fear and fascination as children, naturally assumed that it had always been present in the forests and glens. It became known to everyone as the 'bush bee'. The singular ability to survive those long ocean voyages on 'the smell of an oily rag' meant that the European black bee didn't really need any ongoing help or assistance from humans. All it required was an initial ride, and English missionaries and colonial settlers kindly provided the transport, not just to Australia and New Zealand, but to many of the Pacific Islands as well. It became a feral animal, just like wild pigs and goats.

The missionaries brought honey bees with them for the very liturgical reason that they needed those beeswax candles for church services, although of course the honey would have also been most welcome, particularly with jam and even sugar in short supply. As for the settlers, it was one thing to bring fruit trees like apples and pears to New Zealand, as well as clover to help establish the nutritious pastures for sheep and cows. Once they were planted, however, they needed another important part of that European agricultural ecosystem, an insect to pollinate those new species. With pasture management in New Zealand today becoming more and more dependent on hydrocarbon-based artificial nitrogen fertilisers, we sometimes forget that it was white clover that helped establish and maintain the rotationally grazed, year-round pastoral system that is still the basis of the country's economic prosperity. Settlers may not then have understood that clover 'fixes' nitrogen in the soil, but they were quick to understand the benefits of honey bees. As one eye-witness of the role of honey bees in New Zealand's agricultural development said, 'Before the introduction of the honey bee they had to send over to England every year for the white clover seed, as it did not seed freely here. But by the agency of the bees they are now able to export it.'*

By 1842, honey bee importations had become an organised business, with notices appearing in the *New Zealand Journal* advertising 'Bees for sale; expected from Sydney; orders will be taken for importations to the extent of from 20 to 30 hives.' And Governor Hobson had clearly been impressed by Mary's bees during his stay at Mangungu, since he also now had his own hives.

Cotton devised a complicated system using ice in insulated barrels to keep the bee colonies in those skep hives from perishing during the long voyages, although it is unclear whether it was ever used. More common was the feeding of honey to the hives while on board ship, including the use of glass tubes made especially for the purpose on a journey that brought the first honey bees to Nelson in 1842. In fact, ship's passengers willing to take over such duties were sometimes offered one of the hives upon safe completion of the trip.*

On voyages from England, or later the west coast of the United States, the colonies of honey bees were allowed to fly about while the ships were in port. And in the case of Mary Bumby's skeps, the good ship *James* spent 36 days in Hobart, Tasmania, before proceeding to the Hokianga. Presumably the bees were given free rein to feed on the flowers blooming in what was then called Van Diemen's Land. In another case some years later, the captain arranged to have his ship travelling from California to Australia dock in Honolulu at daybreak, and not leave again before nightfall, allowing the bees on board to visit the exotic flowers of Hawaii for the entire day.*

Picturesque ... but not profitable

In the second half of the nineteenth century, as New Zealand was being changed from a land of forests, scrub and fen, to a patchwork of productive pastures, beekeeping began to develop from a few skeps in the back garden to something more large scale.* As we've seen, Great Barrier Island was arguably the first place with commercial apiaries, but that honour was also claimed by a similar business in Matamata, in the Waikato region of the North Island. Its owner was a man who would change the face of beekeeping in the country.

Isaac Hopkins was an indefatigable champion of the modern methods of beekeeping developed by Langstroth in the United States. He imported the moveable frame hives into New Zealand in 1876 and, like many beekeepers who followed, immediately began constructing them himself. A foundation press soon followed, to make the beeswax sheets embossed with hexagons the bees would use to make comb in the frames. Not all beekeepers followed his lead, however, and *box hives* (bees living in the wooden equivalent of skeps without moveable frames) became very popular, especially since empty butter boxes used in the early years of the dairy industry were easy to come by and very cheap.

Hopkins also popularised a new strain of bee, the Italian bee (*Apis mellifera ligustica*). While the distance between New Zealand and the rest of the world has always made communication difficult, Hopkins was right up with the latest trends, corresponding with beekeepers in Great Britain, the United States and Australia. So when word began to spread about the superior characteristics of this new bee, imported to America by Langstroth in 1874, and into Australia in 1876, Hopkins had to have some of his own.

The Italian bee was everything the German black bee was not. For starters, it was golden yellow, with little black stripes. It was quiet on the combs, while the black bees were prone to run around, and in the case of the queen even hide, no doubt because it proved a successful defence mechanism against the predations of beekeepers cutting combs out of skeps. The Italians were also gentle, and less prone to stinging. Most of all, though, the Italian bee produced prodigious crops of honey. But this did come at some cost. Italian bees were 'hopeful', growing out lots of brood and bees in the spring, regardless of the weather. In New Zealand's changeable climate, however, that sometimes meant that if they weren't managed properly, and even fed, hives could starve to death, especially in the early spring. As a result, European blacks continued to be the feral honey bee of the New Zealand bush, because they didn't need any human assistance, while Italians became the predominant bee kept in hives. Matings between the two strains would occur, however, producing some often very aggressive results, so beekeepers began to rely on specialist queen producers who could supply more pure-bred Italian stock.

Hopkins was also a great populariser. In the 1880s he wrote no fewer than four New Zealand and Australasian beekeeping manuals, began the first beekeeping journal in the Southern Hemisphere, and in 1884 helped in the formation of a New Zealand beekeepers' association. A photograph from the time shows Hopkins, with neatly trimmed white beard, tweed cap and three-piece suit, bending over three straw skeps at an agricultural exposition. A sign mounted in front of the hive makes his feelings clear about the need for modern beekeeping methods. It reads: *Picturesque ... But Not Profitable!* *

Above all else, however, Hopkins was instrumental in helping this newly developed industry survive its first major crisis, one that threatened to bring it to its knees. A bee disease was reported for the first time in the country in 1877. It was called American foul-brood, since it was first observed in the United States, and because it attacked the developing brood of the hive. The dead remains

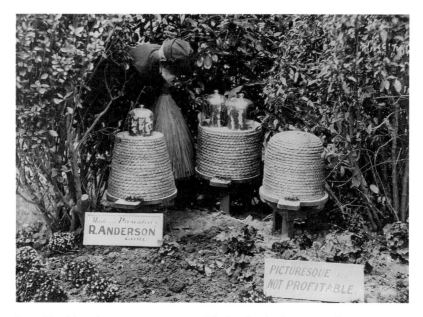

Isaac Hopkins, the man most responsible for developing a sound commercial beekeeping industry in New Zealand and a champion of the use of moveable frame hives. The sign in front of the skeps reads, 'Picturesque … But Not Profitable!'

gave off a noticeably bad smell. Within 10 years the disease had spread to all parts of New Zealand and was being blamed for a 70% reduction in the nation's honey production. While it was only decades later that the cause of the disease was determined to be a honey bee-specific type of bacteria, based on what he had read in overseas publications and his own observations Hopkins became convinced that the only way to effectively deal with the infection was to routinely inspect combs for its presence, and then destroy any diseased material by burning.[†]

To do that, however, beekeepers had to have hives that they could easily disassemble in order to investigate the health of the brood, so a campaign got under way to ensure that all honey bees were kept in moveable frame hives. It took Hopkins more than a

---

[†]   Hopkins had many detractors, and, with the advent of synthetic antibiotics after World War II, beekeeping in many parts of the world started using drug treatment as a standard form of American foulbrood prevention. New Zealand never adopted that method, however, and in recent years, with the development of antibiotic-resistant strains of the disease-causing bacteria, the search/destroy/sterilise/quarantine method first implemented by this far-sighted father of New Zealand commercial beekeeping is now becoming more popular overseas.

decade, but finally in 1905 an Apiaries Act was adopted, and Isaac Hopkins became the country's first Government Apiarist. Not only were those skeps (and box hives) not profitable, they had now become illegal as well.* Beehives also had to be registered, and apiary inspectors were appointed to help beekeepers with disease inspection and bee husbandry, travelling the countryside on government-issued bicycles. The first national census, in 1906, showed that there were 15,000 beekeepers owning just under 75,000 hives.

The house built on one year's honey crop and the 'Infernal' Marketing Board

The weather can make life very difficult for commercial beekeepers in New Zealand. Good spring conditions can see the population of honey bees in a colony increase so rapidly that there just isn't enough space in a two-box hive. The result can be bees hanging in the trees, as the old queen departs with a swarm, leaving behind the remaining bees and a new queen still to hatch from its cell. With inclement weather, on the other hand, the bees begin to starve, and the beekeeper has to visit the hives giving them sugar syrup, or frames of honey that have been kept in the shed over winter for that eventuality.

This latter type of situation was what occurred in Southland one year in the early 1900s. Robert Gibbs was a schoolteacher, but also a beekeeper, and he had finally given up his paying position as headmaster at Tuturau. But the spring weather that year was atrocious, and at the end of January he was still feeding sugar to his hives to keep the bees alive. Luckily the Education Board offered him back a teaching post, but he was only in the job for a week when, as he says, 'Conditions changed overnight. So heavy was the honey flow from the clover that one's boots became sticky when walking through the pasture', and the bottom of his wife's long skirt became wet with nectar when she went for an evening's stroll. Gibbs produced 14 tons from 150 hives (85 kilograms per hive), packed it all into 2-pound tins, and exported it to England, receiving 1 shilling per pound. He used the money to construct a home, which he christened 'Beeswing'. The name was outlined in a beautiful lead-light window above the door. Ever after, he took great pride in telling visitors that it was a house built on one year's honey crop.*

But as with all agricultural production, particularly when you're a country with a small population a long way from your export markets, it's very easy to have too much of a good thing. Moveable frame hives, control of American foulbrood, and those Italian bees helped beekeepers begin to produce more honey than the local population could eat, even though New Zealanders were (and continue to be) some of the largest consumers of honey per capita in the world. Initially it was the beekeepers' association itself that started to act as a clearinghouse for honey exports, since its members complained about low prices on the domestic market, and the need to clear existing stocks so that they didn't further depress prices. And clearly stories like that of Robert Gibbs opened up beekeepers' eyes to what could be achieved if they could just get their honey overseas.

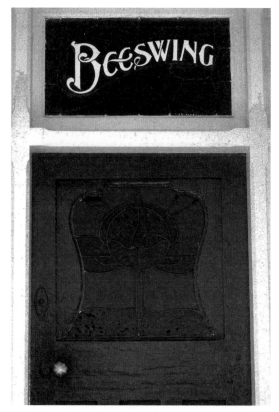

The lead-light window over the door of 'Beeswing', the house Robert Gibbs built on the proceeds of one year's honey crop in the early 1900s.

Co-operative marketing of agricultural products has been around since almost the dawn of industrial agriculture, and it has been a feature of the New Zealand economy in various forms since the small Otago Peninsula Co-operative Cheese Factory Co. was started near Dunedin in 1871. The reason for *co-operatives* is fairly straightforward. Markets for farmers' products can be very far away, and it's quite easy for the distributors and sellers of those products to play individual farmers off against each other. When you are far away from the dinner plate, and communications can be as slow as a boat, it is very difficult to know what the going rate is for your lamb or your butter. Co-operatives help ensure that the playing field is a lot more level, since groups of producers carry a lot more clout. Government *marketing boards*, on the other hand, became necessary in times of depressed agricultural prices, since the guarantee of the state was needed to back payments to suppliers. They were seen as necessary to protect the livelihoods of farmers and others in rural communities.

The same arguments were thought to apply to honey. Especially in high-production years in New Zealand, there was just too much honey for the local market to absorb. And for an owner/operator (and most commercial operators try to keep their bees as well as process their product) getting over to the United Kingdom or Germany, the largest markets for that honey, would be impossible. It was also very difficult to obtain finance, since of course beekeepers have their assets mostly tied up in beehives. So, like many other farmers, they looked to the government to assist them in exporting.

For its part, the government felt that it had a role to play, too, since it wanted to ensure the largest amount of foreign exchange was brought back to the country for whatever it sold abroad. So the model that was followed was *export licensing*; namely, that a government-assisted organisation would have exclusive rights to exports. In exchange for that monopoly, however, the organisation would be required to buy any and all of the produce from farmers that was suitable for sale. A minimum price was set at the beginning of the season, proceeds of sales were put into a pool, and at the end of the year, if all went well, a bonus pay-out was distributed. Thus was formed the Meat Board, the Dairy

Board (which eventually amalgamated with many small dairy co-operatives to become Fonterra), the Apple and Pear Marketing Board, and the Kiwifruit Marketing Board (now known as Zespri). In the case of honey, there was the legislated Honey Control Board, with all export honey handled by the Honey Producers' Association. That group went bankrupt in the 1930s, thanks to bad debts from its British agents. Then in 1938 came the Internal — or 'Infernal', as they called it on the Barrier and elsewhere — Marketing Department, a true government marketing board, followed by the Honey Marketing Authority (the HMA) in 1953. In each case , these entities had the authority to buy and market honey locally, and to control its export.

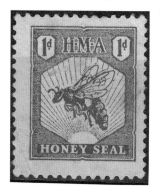

Stamp duty, part of the funding mechanism the New Zealand Honey Marketing Authority used to finance sales of both domestic and export honey. The stamps, which had to be fixed to retail honey packs, are now a valuable collectors' item.

There were a couple of problems with the model so far as honey was concerned, however. One was that, unlike for dairy produce or meat, there wasn't an in-built need for a central organisation to process and preserve the product. If honey is under 20% moisture when extracted and kept in a closed container, it just doesn't spoil. So any beekeeper could also be a processor and packer, selling the finished item direct to the retailer in a handy serving container. The other problem was that New Zealand produced some 'interesting' honeys. Some — rewarewa, kamahi, pohutukawa, rata and manuka — were from native floral sources that didn't exist anywhere else in the world. And others — honeydew, thyme and heather — were honeys that were well known in Europe, but completely foreign to the established tastes of New Zealanders. These honeys could certainly be exported, but they needed to be handled separately, and not that much was produced, and not consistently enough, to be able to easily develop a market overseas. It was much easier for the marketing boards to flog the big bulk honeys, which fit into the standards commonly being used around the world. Number one was colour, and the lighter the better. After that it was just a matter of the honey being bland enough that it didn't upset the taste buds of the vast majority of consumers.

So beginning in 1915, and carrying right through to the HMA, the government set grade standards, and used professional honey graders to ensure there was no fraud or even favouritism shown to suppliers. Once the graders had done their work, the honey of each colour (extra white, white, light amber, amber, dark amber) was combined into bulk tanks and blended in an attempt to create 'standard' lines. Pohutukawa might be blended with rata and clover to make light-coloured blends, while darker honeys like rewarewa were often combined with the stronger-tasting kamahi. The white honeys were *table grade*, and fetched the best price. Some of it was sold on the local market, and the remainder exported. The ambers were relegated to industrial uses, and hopefully sold either abroad or at home to bakeries and food manufacturers.

For anyone who wasn't around at the time, it seems a strange system indeed. But it fit with what everyone thought were international requirements. If it had been wine, it would be the equivalent of trying to make as much table-grade plonk as possible, while turning stronger flavoured Chardonnays and Rieslings into vinegar.

A most peculiar honey

The problem with manuka honey was that it just didn't fit into the system. As we saw earlier, even in Auckland at the turn of the twentieth century it was fetching half the price of clover. And it didn't get any better. During World War I the Honey Producers' Association managed to find sales for it in Britain, where its agent sold it as 'New Zealand heather'. Both manuka and heather had one thing in common: they were hard to remove from the comb. But then the New Zealand Agriculture Department announced that there was no heather in the country (and at this point they were right). So a highly lucrative market, albeit one based on a bit of false advertising, was lost.

Manuka honey continued to be purchased by the Internal Marketing Department, but only as an assistance to beekeepers who for one reason or another ended up producing it. In 1951 — at about the same time that Great Barrier Island beekeeper Les Blackwell vowed never again to sell to the 'Infernal' Marketing

Department — discussion at the National Beekeepers' Association centred on the marketing of manuka honey. Conference records reported that: 'During the past season unusual quantities of dark honeys were produced in northern areas and it was becoming evident that in future manuka honey would be very difficult to sell on a normal market.' It was 'definitely unsuitable for blending and when outlets can be found for it ... the return is very disappointing'.* The Honey Control Board itself said that it could buy it from beekeepers only 'by means of a subsidy from the returns for high-grade honey'. The conference therefore supported the opinion of the Honey Marketing Committee that: 'Manuka honey should not be included in the pool, but should be marketed separately, by agreement with the supplier, to the best advantage possible.'

The message was clear. In an address to the same association two years later, the Director of the Horticulture Division of the Department of Agriculture put it bluntly: 'Manuka honey cannot be clarified or blended with other honey by the usual methods. Because of this difficulty, beekeepers are not being encouraged to produce this type of honey. However, where it is impossible for a beekeeper to move from a manuka area the honey produced must be handled.'* Plans were therefore drawn up for special equipment to deal with the unique nature of the honey, including how to successfully remove it from the comb without cutting it from the frames and pressing it, as Les Blackwell described beekeepers doing on Great Barrier Island. There was even an attempt by government scientists to filter the honey to the point that it lost most of its colour and flavour in the hopes that 'the resulting product (invert sugar) will find a demand for manufacturing purposes'.*

The 'difficulty' the Director of the Horticulture Division was referring to is something that, along with heather, makes manuka unique in the world of honeys. It's a characteristic called *thixotropy*, also known by the delightful term physicists use — they say it displays 'non-Newtonian' properties. Put simply, what that means is if you take a spoonful of either of these honeys in a warmed liquid form and turn the spoon upside down, the honey doesn't drip off in a steady stream. It more or less stays there like a dollop of jelly, defying Sir Isaac Newton's famous gravity.

Jelly is the apt description, because, just like the agar that cooks use to make a liquid set, what keeps these honeys in suspension are special proteins that with their long strands tangle through each other, binding the moisture, glucose and fructose that make up the honey into a sort of jumble of intertwining nets.

The discovery of these proteins in both heather and manuka honeys was made in the early 1950s, and with it a possible solution to the problem of extracting the honey without having to press it, comb and all. If you agitate the honey you break up the chains, and it starts behaving the way all other honeys do, dripping off spoons and spinning out of combs. Eventually, however, the proteins reform themselves, and turn into a gel again.

New Zealand scientists worked out a series of methods to help beekeepers remove manuka honey from their combs. One involved using a board with handles on one side and lots of small nails on the other. It was found that if you pushed the board (called a *pricker pad*) repeatedly onto the face of the comb, the nails would *excite* the honey, and allow it to be spun out. A similar device used a set of little knives that, while meant to stir up the honey, also tended to tear the comb to shreds. The process was both messy and time-consuming, not to mention very tiring for the person manning the board. For that reason — and the fact that thixotropy

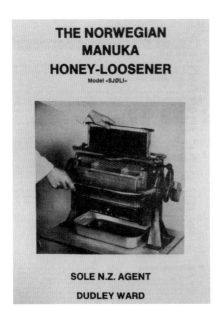

THE NORWEGIAN MANUKA HONEY-LOOSENER
Model «SJØLI»

SOLE N.Z. AGENT

DUDLEY WARD

The Norwegian 'Honningløsner' that solved the problem of how to extract thixotropic manuka honey efficiently.

also made manuka honey very difficult to strain — as late as 1962 the official New Zealand beekeeping manual 'warned against the establishment of apiaries close to manuka areas if it is intended to produce extracted honey for ordinary trade purposes'.*

The final solution to the problem, as it turned out, came from the other side of the world. The Norwegians, like beekeepers elsewhere in the Baltic region and those on the Scottish moors, produced heather honey, and of course it was thixotropic, too. So they designed something called the 'Honningløsner'. (If you sound it out you'll find there's at least one Norwegian word that's easy to understand!) The machine consisted of a solid metal frame that sat on a bench. The frame held two plates, one on either side, and mounted on those plates were sets of tiny fibreglass and nylon needles, held in place with stainless steel springs. All the beekeeper had to do was place a frameful of honey in the machine and pull a level up and down. The plates would push towards the comb, the needles would pierce the cappings, and the springs would move the needles in and out, loosening the honey, but hopefully not damaging the wax hexagons that hold the honey on the frame. It was then a simple matter of putting the combs into a normal honey extractor, turning it on, and letting centrifugal force take over from there.

The honey loosener is still the system used today with manuka honey, although crafty New Zealand engineers have designed similar machines that are so fully automated that no one has to even move the handles by hand. As for filtering the extracted honey, especially to remove the little bits of wax capping that are dislodged by the needles moving in and out, that problem was solved by creating a barrel encased in screen mesh which rotated as the honey was pumped into it. Vanes in the barrel would keep the honey agitated, and clean honey would drip out the sides.*

Site honey and honesty boxes
While the technical challenges posed by manuka honey were eventually sorted out, there was still the problem of trying to find a sale for the product. The Honningløsner was expensive, and if you couldn't get a reasonable price for your crop you couldn't afford one. So beekeepers employed other strategies.

Sometimes a beekeeper in almost any part of the country might get caught out, failing to follow that warning in the official government beekeeping manual to avoid keeping hives near bush where manuka might be found. That wasn't always as simple as it might sound, however, especially if a new apiary was set out and the stand of manuka was over a hill or deep in a valley. The beekeeper might not be able to see it from the road, but the bees certainly had no trouble finding the manuka when it was in full bloom. In such cases, a common approach was to keep the honey in the shed and use it to feed back to hives early the next spring. If you blew it, however, and ended up with more manuka honey than you could possibly use, a phone call was sometimes made to a fellow beekeeper down the line. A deal was struck, and full boxes of manuka honey were exchanged for the equivalent number of empty, extracted combs. You really did give the stuff away.

For beekeepers in areas where manuka was a predominant species, on the other hand, such as in the far north of the North Island, finding manuka-free areas to keep bees often wasn't on the cards. Murray Reid, who these days follows on in the proud tradition of Isaac Hopkins as Government Apiarist (his official title is National Manager — Apiculture), helped pay for his university education in the late 1960s by working for three summers for Palmer Apiaries in Dargaville, Northland.

The local area had both large tracts of manuka, as well as mixed farming, so the strategy that was used involved producing an early crop of manuka honey, followed by a later flow from pasture species such as clover, buttercup and even pennyroyal (that minty herb that had gone wild, and which had become a feature in drought-prone pastures in the north). Much of the manuka crop would be stored in the shed and kept for feed. Production would often be so good, however, that they had more than they could use for the purpose. So Murray remembers spending days in the honey house, using an early model of an automatic honey-loosener with a single row of nails that damaged the combs, and then putting them through the extractor, generally with very mixed results. You could tell that not all the honey had been removed as soon as you lifted the frames out of the machine.

The honey itself was packed into 4-gallon tins (each holding 28 kilograms), for sale to the Honey Marketing Authority at about half the price of clover-type honey, as well as in 1- and 2-pound waxed cardboard containers for local retail sales. Manuka honey was often given to the farmers who provided the small amount of space, usually at the back of their properties, where beehives were placed. This *site honey*, as it was called, has always been a welcome addition to the larder of rural families throughout New Zealand, and as Murray says, many of the farmers seemed to prefer the taste of the stronger, darker manuka honey to the light clover that was sold in the grocery stores in town.

The Dargaville beekeeping business also sold honey directly to the public from a small stall with an 'honesty box' (where the purchaser put their coins) at the side of the road. Again, judging by the many repeat customers, there was a demand for the product, at least in the countryside, if not from bulk honey-traders overseas.

A long-time beekeeper named Malcolm Haines also remembers what it used to be like in the Far North with little but manuka around to produce a honey crop. His father, Bill, virtually pioneered beekeeping at the very tip of the North Island, moving to Kaitaia after World War II. Malcolm especially recalls the flats in the Ahipara district, which these days are cattle and dairy farms, being at that time nothing but stands of manuka as far as the eye could see.

The Haines family also kept manuka honey for feed, but Malcolm says they did have plenty of sales for their product. They made a regular delivery run to grocery stores throughout the north, and also at times delivered surplus crop in 60-pound tins and later 200-kilogram drums to the Honey Marketing Authority depot in Parnell in Auckland. The honey never achieved the top price, being graded well down the colour scale, but the HMA was still an outlet when push came to shove.

The Haines were also entrepreneurs, however, and since they were in the sub-tropical north, with the earliest springs in New Zealand, and a honey crop that also finished and was extracted months earlier than those further south, they diversified their business to produce queen bees for sale throughout the country, and even *package bees*. Packages are artificial swarms of bees without any comb, which are put in a screened cage about the size of a breadbox, and shipped complete with a sugar syrup feeder and a newly mated queen. Package bees were very popular in the western United States, where tens of thousands were transported each spring by truck from California to the rich honey-production areas of the Canadian prairies. Malcolm eventually worked together with other like-minded beekeepers in New Zealand to transport these packages from the New Zealand autumn to the Canadian spring in the air-conditioned holds of passenger jets.*

Malcolm also had foresight. At a special conference on honey marketing held in Taupo in 1974, just as calls for change in the way honey was exported began to stir within the industry, he gave a speech in which he said that, while many beekeepers were turned off by the production of dark honeys, and thixotropic manuka honey in particular, and others regarded it only as a feed source, in his opinion it was a good honey to market and its demand would certainly increase.* No doubt many in the audience would have scoffed at the statement, especially given the good prices the HMA was achieving for clover honey, both domestically and overseas. As we'll see, however, Malcolm most certainly had the last laugh.

The big honey stoush

Centralised marketing and export controls of honey may have made sense, especially if you were a commercial beekeeper in the sparsely populated South Island, produced clover honey that graded out at *white* or even *extra-white*, and got even more points for it because it was *delicate* on the flavour chart. It was going to be very hard to sell your honey yourself, given the large amounts you could produce, and no doubt the scarcity of customers driving past your door. It was far easier to just extract the honey (no Honningløsner required), put it into drums, and phone for a transport truck. As for the managers of the Honey Marketing Authority, it was also a pretty simple matter to offer it for sale on the international market. The big buyers in Europe knew all about clover, since it was the most common honey produced around the world. In fact, a company in the United Kingdom called Kimptons was quite happy to take almost all of it, along with even some of the darker and less delicate flavoured grades (at a lower price, of course).

Colonel Kimpton, the head of the firm, would come out to New Zealand every year, wine and dine the managers and beekeeper directors, then sign a contract for another year. It was a sweet deal, almost all around. There was just one slight problem. The regulations that controlled the HMA and honey exports did allow for a couple of exceptions. Comb honey, a product some people regard as the ultimate type of honey to eat on toast, couldn't be graded because it hadn't been extracted. As well, honeydew from the South Island was starting to develop as a honey source, and for some reason it didn't qualify either. Finally, if you packed your own retail lines of honey, and made sure it met the export standards for honey, you could try to sell that overseas, too.

There was no issue with that last commodity, however, at least so far as the HMA was concerned. It argued quite forcefully in an information circular to beekeeper suppliers that, while the export market for retail packs could not be ignored, 'The total quantity involved is so small as to have no significant effect on returns to producers.' Packaging and especially freight costs were too high, glass jars would break in transit, and quality plastic wasn't available because of import controls. Lastly, the big international players were just too strong, and with New Zealand's fluctuating production of most honeys other than clover, the HMA contended we couldn't guarantee enough supply.*

Comb honey was selling well overseas, however, and to some places quite different from our traditional markets. The Middle East was experiencing a boom in consumer spending brought on by oil exports, and Arabs in particular loved comb honey. How could they not, given that the Prophet Mohammed himself recommended it?

And so a small man (but only in stature) who owned a very big beekeeping company, Percy Berry of Arataki Honey, travelled abroad to secure contracts for comb honey for himself and a number of his fellow beekeepers in the North Island. He saw how honey from around the world, including New Zealand, was being packaged and marketed in Europe and elsewhere, and he came back home determined to bring about a change.

There followed some of the most turbulent times in the history of beekeeping in New Zealand, with remits flying back and forth at the National Beekeepers' Association conferences, and at one point nearly a few fists flying as well. It became something of a North Island–South Island split, although not entirely. Eventually Percy got himself elected as chairman of the Honey Marketing Authority, and a compromise solution worked out between all parties was finally reached. The HMA would be abolished, and in its place would be a honey producers' co-operative, centred in the South Island. It would retain at least some of the authority's assets (with the remainder placed in a research and promotion trust), and would continue to produce honey for the New Zealand market under the famous Holland's brand.* The co-op would also trade honey internationally, but would no longer have monopoly control. Beekeeping had, in effect, become one of the first agricultural industries in the country to voluntarily open up free trade of its products internationally.

Overseas, in the United States, they were definitely moving in the opposite direction. The federal government created a honey price stabilisation programme under the auspices of the Commodity Credit Corporation. This agency lent beekeepers money at the time they produced their crop, using the honey as collateral, and then let them buy it back later on in the year once the production glut was over and prices had hopefully stabilised.* The result was a honey mountain (or perhaps when it got too hot, a honey lake). It sometimes became a subsidy by another name, particularly when the value of the loan exceeded the buy-back price. Many thousands of pounds of American honey would remain for long periods in rented warehouses, often owned by the beekeepers themselves.

The European Community has been much more up-front. Today, beekeepers' incomes are directly supported under the Common Agriculture Programme. As well, they receive technical assistance and sometimes even direct payments. Part of the argument for these extra support programmes to beekeepers is that there needs to be a recognition of the pollination their bees provide to both crops and wild plants throughout the countryside, most often without any other form of payment.*

In New Zealand, on the other hand, there are no subsidies for any part of agriculture, including beekeeping. Even basic services like technical advice, disease control and export certification are strictly 'user pays'. Some might argue that what happened with honey in New Zealand was a free-market revolution, while it is likely that others will point out that it was simply the result of improvements in travel and communication which finally made it possible to access the information needed to make a real market work for the benefit of the seller, not just the traders overseas. Regardless, without it the fortunes of manuka honey might never have changed.*

Although not many people could clearly see it at the time, bee-keeping in the country had literally turned on its axis, from South Island to North Island, from export controls to entrepreneurialism, and from honey as only a food to something a lot more powerful. The scene was set. All that was needed was a cast of players and the right sort of energy. As it turned out, it was a marketing dynamo of a man, quite new to honey, who was about to provide the spark.

Four

THE PRESS RELEASE
THAT GREW LEGS

Late in November 1991, a press release was sent out. The internet and email were only just coming into their own in New Zealand, so the document was faxed to the various newspapers, magazines, and radio and TV outlets throughout the country. As a piece of prose it perhaps wasn't all that punchy and hard-hitting, at least when judged by the sort of journalistic standards that can sometimes see writing pitched at 30-second attention spans and the reading level of 12-year-olds.

In fact, the copy went on for more than two pages, and mentioned — along with a certain senior lecturer at the University of Waikato and his discovery about an unusual honey — a range of topics, including stressed executives, stomach ulcers, Hippocrates, and those Mesopotamian clay tablets (the first 'written' records of honey used as a medicine). It also included, however, a quite remarkable paragraph on the use of honey as a wound dressing, and a quote to finish by that senior lecturer: '"It is clear," says Dr Peter Molan, "that manuka honeys have qualities that surpass any other honeys."'*

The joke was that it must have been a slow news day, because quite quickly Peter's telephone started ringing off the hook. And it continued well past the end of the normal media cycle. The press release certainly didn't become tomorrow's fish wrapper, that's for sure. It had, as they say in media circles, 'grown legs'. It seemed as though journalists everywhere in the world wanted to know about this honey from New Zealand with an interesting name, and its even more remarkable properties. Could it actually kill disease-causing bacteria? And was it really possible to treat burns and wounds successfully with something that was, let's face it, a food?

On and on it went. The press release kept appearing in media around the world, even four years later, almost verbatim. And Peter received requests for interviews from some of the most unusual places. The most improbable, he recalls, was from *Cosmopolitan* magazine in the United States. With articles on topics such as how to tell your boyfriend what you want in the bedroom, and the latest news on lip gloss and foundation makeup, it wasn't exactly the sort of publication you would think was interested in a new scientific discovery in microbiology, or even woundcare research. But Peter reckons *Cosmopolitan*'s reporters and staff were some of the most professional and well-prepared he's ever dealt with.*

The person responsible for that press release was Bill Floyd, from Blenheim. And, believe it or not, the reason he sent it off from his fax machine turns out to have a direct link to the dissolution of the Honey Marketing Authority, and the effects that freeing up honey exports were now having on New Zealand beekeeping.

It is a story of both industry co-operation and strong competition which in the end would put manuka honey and New Zealand bee-keeping firmly on the map. A most peculiar and very neglected honey was about to become famous around the world.

An industry with a plan

In 1988, a former beekeeping advisor with the Ministry of Agriculture was managing a beekeeping operation in the Far North. With all his experience he should have been well placed to follow recommendations made in the past about not putting his apiaries near manuka scrub. It was a very good spring, however, and his hope was that the hives he had just put in three new apiaries near the bushline would sit quietly, and be ready for kiwifruit pollination when November rolled around. Instead, the bees in those hives brought in massive crops of manuka honey.

Rather than keep the honey for feed, the decision was taken to extract it. So the beekeeper and his staff went through the ordeal of hand-pricking all the combs and putting them through their extractor, which was only designed to handle honeys like clover that didn't stick so hard to the frames. The resulting honey filled three barrels (just under a tonne), but the problems really began when the beekeeper tried to find someone to buy it. He called friends throughout the industry, and even food-manufacturing companies further south. They sympathised with his predicament, but all said they couldn't help. Finally one kind fellow called back. He said he could at least take the honey off the beekeeper's hands, and pay for transport of the full drums down to his depot. He would then look for a buyer on his own, and send the money back if and when one was found. That beekeeper, I must confess, was yours truly. And I have no idea what happened to the honey. The company I worked for, which owned kiwifruit orchards and packhouses, sold all the beehives the next year and I moved on.

But what my story does show is that the New Zealand bee-keeping industry wasn't somehow magically transformed overnight by export deregulation. In fact, the evidence seems to suggest that prices for manuka honey in particular may have fallen away after the HMA ceased trading, probably because those most interested in exporting New Zealand honey in a private capacity still found it much easier to sell lighter and more delicate-tasting honey types. Before 1982, at least the HMA would take manuka honey off beekeepers' hands, since it had a requirement to do so by law. Once the authority disappeared, not that many people wanted to know.

As for the domestic market, as we've seen from some of the beekeeper stories the darker bush honeys like manuka did find at least a bit of acceptance, especially in some of the provincial areas. But as for the more urban consumers who generally bought their honey at the grocery stores, their taste preference was most definitely for clover honey, since this was the predominate honey on the market, and while it could be exported it was still being retailed domestically at a fairly low price.

The sale of honey is an example of a classic market economy. For starters, there are few impediments to entrance into the market. Capital costs — in the form of production, extraction and processing — are low (although not as low as they once were in New Zealand, due to increased regulation by the country's Food Safety Authority). At the same time, honey doesn't spoil if handled properly, and doesn't need any special treatment or manufacturing. It is also easy to find buyers for the product, either through supermarkets and other food outlets, or via sales at the beekeeper's door. What all this means, of course, is that there are lots of wholesalers of honey products in the market, with little capital backing, and so their selling behaviour is driven by the demands of their cash flow. The result, as can be expected in a classic market, is low prices compared with the cost of production. Most beekeepers in such a situation can't hold on to the honey they produce for too long.

As with most markets, information and communication is never fully adequate, but the beekeeper grapevine is well established, and

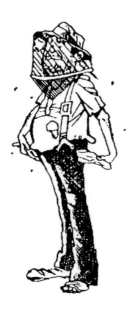

as a result prices tend to be set by the softest sellers. In the past, the prices were depressed even further by what became a well-established practice of supermarkets in New Zealand of using honey as a *loss leader*, a discounted food item that stores use to lure customers in. Such prices can sometimes provide the impetus for soft sellers to try to match what is in effect a cost price offered by the supermarket, since the soft sellers are sometimes unaware of the wholesale price that was obtained by their competitor who supplied the store.

The 'poor beekeeper' cartoon that appeared in the beekeepers' association newsletter in 1989, just as that organisation took its first tentative steps to create a Marketing Committee and a honey promotional plan.

It seems hard to believe now, but back in the 1980s there was significant concern being expressed by the National Beekeepers' Association about the ability of many of its commercial members to remain in business. As late as 1989 a cartoon was printed in one of the association's publications that showed a beekeeper wearing his veil over an old hat. His shirt and pants had patches, and he was pulling out his pockets to show he didn't have any cash. For many of the readers, the cartoon was likely to have been more poignant than humorous.

For its part, the government certainly wasn't helping matters. The economic liberalism that became orthodoxy during the era resulted over time in a change to 'user pays' for beekeeping extension, research, and finally disease control services. Eventually the policy makers in Wellington, and their 'Yes, Minister' politicians decided to do away even with Isaac Hopkins's original Apiaries Act, which with some modifications had served the beekeeping industry so well for almost a century. In order to continue on with the sort of American foulbrood control systems Hopkins had seen as vitally important, the National Beekeepers' Association was forced to come up with something called a Pest Management Strategy (PMS) under a new Biosecurity Act.

The Act, which had never really been tested thoroughly to solve some of its drafting issues, was meant to allow agricultural industries to create their own disease control programmes, provided of course they paid for them themselves. In the case of the National Beekeepers' Association, it struggled through the process with a dedicated group of volunteers, attempting to meet demanding deadlines, and acting as a guinea pig to see how the Act would work. The government eventually had to pass an amendment that ran to 71 pages and 116 clauses, about two-thirds the size of the original Act.

In the end, the beekeepers' association got what it needed, and its PMS became one of only two national programmes developed by industries themselves. But the whole process, which took years to complete, left a bad taste in the mouths of many beekeepers. Government in New Zealand was no longer seen as the helpmate of beekeeping that it once was.*

Faced with all these sorts of problem, the beekeeping industry decided to do something that might seem obvious, but back then was a remarkably innovative idea: it came up with a plan.

The astute and congenial president of the National Beekeepers' Association at the time, Allen McCaw, from the small settlement of Milburn in the far south of the South Island, convened a series of meetings, and brought together a number of like-minded beekeepers from around the country. There was certainly some enmity in the organisation left over from the HMA battles. But there was also a remarkable level of support, perhaps created by that very same co-operative approach to honey marketing that had gone on for so many years.

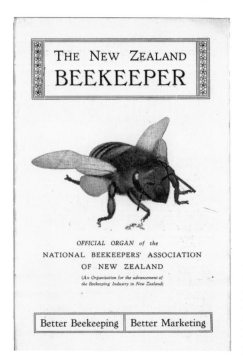

A vintage (1940) copy of *The New Zealand Beekeeper*, the journal of the National Beekeepers' Association, with the association's motto ('Better Beekeeping, Better Marketing') prominently displayed.

Using a set of processes that at the time was beginning to take hold in New Zealand businesses (as well as in the Ministry of Agriculture), Allen and his colleagues carried out a SWOT analysis (Strengths/Weakness/Opportunities/Threats), created some goals (one of which had for many years already been the association's motto: 'Better Beekeeping, Better Marketing'), and a set of quite specific objectives that were reviewed on a regular basis. One of those 'Management by Objectives' was to set up a marketing committee, with the express purpose of doing as much as they could to increase the price of honey. As it turned out, the committee eventually succeeded beyond anyone's wildest dreams (although it's very doubtful if it ever got the credit it deserved).*

The future of honey … Is there life after toast?

'The innate goodness of honey is its number one competitive advantage.'

'If honey is marketed the way it should be, consumers will seek it out in products the way they now do for oat bran.'

'When honey is battling for breakfast table space with jam and marmalade, and that's the only time people think about it, you are vulnerable to it being treated as one big thick tablespoon of homogeneous product ... a price-sensitive commodity line.'

'If you negotiate with a food chain and they sense you <u>have</u> to sell, you'll be lucky to recover the cost of your time and packaging, let alone the honey inside. The chains aren't to blame; they're just doing their job. But you as an industry are to blame if you split yourselves up and shoot each other in the foot.'

'Most New Zealand agricultural-based industries have been production-led. We have taken our superb and unique natural resources and produced milk and meat and honey and more ... and then looked for people to buy what we've produced. That's where marketing comes in. It is, of course, common sense to provide what people <u>really</u> want, but it's amazing how often it isn't done.'

These and other similarly pithy statements were part of the address Bill Floyd gave to the National Beekeepers' Association conference in 1991. Attired in a natty suit, with an amazing floral tie, and with his bright-red beard and bushy moustache setting off his balding head, he electrified his audience. It is unlikely that beekeepers — more used to spending very long and often quite hot days out in the paddocks blowing smoke at bees, wielding their all-purpose hive tools, and worrying about what the weather was going to bring — had ever heard anything like it. Bill was someone from outside of the industry with a unique perspective who wasn't afraid to shoot from the hip, and no one had ever addressed a New Zealand beekeeping industry conference that way before.

Bill Floyd had been asked to speak to the gathering by a local member of the Honey Marketing Committee. As he tells it, he pretty much accepted the offer on a whim. His company was involved in marketing contracts with other food businesses, but the more he looked into honey, as he says, 'The more it turned me on.'

The title of the talk was 'Honey, Sweeter Than Wine ...', but he realised after he got deeper into the subject that it should have been, 'The Future for Honey ... Is There Life After Toast?' The answer, he declared, was an emphatic 'Yes!' And looking his audience straight in the eye, he told them, 'It could be surprisingly profitable.'*

The hope of the conference organiser was that beekeepers would stand up and be counted once Bill completed his speech, and maybe pass a resolution that he should be hired to take his ideas further. But everyone seemed to be sitting on their hands. Then a man named Steve Olds stood up. Steve was also from outside the beekeeping industry, and was in fact the owner of a company called Tecpak that produced containers for the developing green-lipped mussel industry in New Zealand. But Steve had fallen in love with honey, too, and so much enjoyed his contact with the local beekeepers who came to buy his packaging materials that he started attending the national conferences. Steve gave a short speech, something about needing to help the industry take advantage of its amazing potential, and then donated $1000 to help launch Bill's work, challenging others to do the same. The ball was rolling, and Bill Floyd wasn't going to let it stop.

The taste of honey, the taste of wine

Imagine, if you will, that people treated honey the same way they did wine. In New Zealand that would mean the many wonderful floral types would have the same sort of terminology used to describe them as is the norm for Sauvignon Blanc, Chardonnay, Pinot Noir and Cabernet. Kamahi — that bush species that produced a honey often only used by bakeries — would be described as 'intense and musky, with a clean, rich finish.' Pohutukawa — the honey from the 'Kiwi Christmas tree' that was given as a gift to King George V — would have a 'salty, almost seaweed aroma, but pleasant, and tasting like sweet butterscotch'. And thyme honey — from the amazingly strong-smelling herb that had taken over parts of Central Otago —would be described as 'very aromatic, with a deep resinous flavour'.

And then there's honeydew. Most New Zealanders have never tasted it. But it you have ever driven from Nelson at the top of the South Island, through the Buller Gorge to the West Coast, you most certainly would have seen the trees that produce it. They are the native species called mountain beech (*Nothofagus solandri*), a tree very different from the beech trees of the Northern

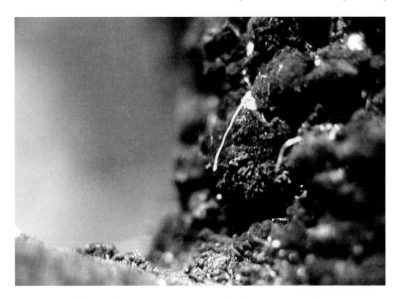

The tiny 'whisker' of a scale insect embedded in the trunk of a mountain beech (*Nothfagus solandri*). The whisker will hold tiny droplets of honeydew collected by bees, wasps and native birds.

Hemisphere, but with a relative in Chile, on the other side of the Pacific Ocean from New Zealand. What makes these trees so different, at least in this part of the country, is that their trunks are absolutely pitch black. You need to stop and examine them more closely, however, to work out the cause. The blackness isn't the bark; it's thick layers of a type of moss-like sooty mould, a fungus that lives exclusively on the sugary sap of the tree that drips out of little hairs protruding from the bark. Each hair is attached to a scale insect that exists nowhere else in the world. The pinkish-coloured *instars* (the plump, stationary stage) embed themselves into the tree, and feed on the sap of the tree flowing just below that bark. But there is so much sap, and the instars are so small, that the insect *exudes* (a nicer-sounding word than *excretes*) the excess out along that hair.

The sap provides food for an entire ecosystem, from bellbirds with their evocative call, right down to minute organisms living in the sooty mould. But honey bees love the sugary substance as well, and they forage for drops of it hanging from the hairs of those scale insects, in much the same way they would collect nectar from flowers. The honey they produce is dark amber in colour, and to use wine connoisseurs' terminology, has a 'musky, mineral and citrus aroma, with a complex, treacly flavour tasting of Christmas cake'. It's called honeydew because that is the generalised name given to honey produced anywhere in the world that comes from insect secretions, the most famous example being from aphids feeding on fir trees in the Black Forest of Germany. In the case of mountain beech honeydew, however, it is more like the New Zealand version of maple syrup — it's just that the bees do most of the work of collection and conversion, rather than ruddy Canadians dressed in red-checked overcoats and snowshoes.*

It was Bill Floyd who helped come up with these and other descriptions of the smells and tastes of New Zealand honeys (what he called 'wine prose'), using the services of food technologists who were expert in the field. He said he just couldn't get over how many unique honeys were produced in New Zealand, and the intensely different characteristics they had.* To get the ideas, all he had to do was drive down the road and visit a couple of wineries in the nearby Marlborough region. New Zealand wine certainly wasn't a commodity, and there was no reason the country's honey had to be either.

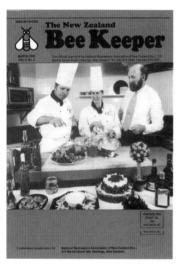

Bill Floyd (right) worked with Denis Taylor and Emily Cross at the Christchurch Polytechnic to encourage chefs throughout the country to develop special dishes using New Zealand's unique range of honeys.

With the help of the Marketing Committee he did tastings of the honeys with food writers, worked with culinary people to create innovative recipes and food products (including a delicious range of honey-flavoured ice creams), and helped incorporate the product as an ingredient in the training of young chefs. A New Zealand honey food and ingredient advisory service was established, and Bill and his wife, Sandee, were even asked to work with the American honey industry. A substantial grant from the US Honey Board for research into American honeys used New Zealand honeys as the benchmark, allowing work to be carried out on the bioactivities of honeys back home, and beekeeping industries in both countries benefited from the deal.

But that was all in the future. The first thing Bill did, almost a year before the beekeepers' association even managed to create a funding mechanism for a fully-fledged honey marketing programme based on a levy of 50 cents per hive, was to start publicising the work of Peter Molan and the special antibacterial properties of manuka honey he had discovered. Looking back, Bill recalls, 'I had heard about this chap up in Hamilton, Peter Molan, and we went up there and talked with him about his research. It had actually been published for some time, but nothing had really come of it. So we decided to use the media to help let people know.' And that's how the famous press release came about.

As to why the publicity had such an amazing effect, Bill reckons that there is an almost magical aspect to the relationship between honey bees and humans. 'Humankind does have something about bees and honey. It's there from the very earliest days. Manuka honey gave us a new way of appreciating one of the great foods and earliest medicines in our world.'

And by the way — just in case you're wondering — according to the New Zealand Honey Sensory Profiles datasheet, manuka honey has a fragrance of 'catmint and heather, with a mineral, slightly bitter and barley sugar flavour'.

The rise of the honey entrepreneurs

People were talking about manuka honey, and they started looking for it in the stores. What was needed was for it no longer to be sold bulk to bakeries or food manufacturers, and if it was put into retail containers, not blended with other honeys like rewarewa and kamahi and labelled 'bush blend'. And — who knows? — if things went well, maybe beekeepers could even start purposely moving their hives into areas where manuka grew.

Several of the more famous names in New Zealand beekeeping took up the manuka challenge. There were the Berrys of Arataki Honey, then the largest beekeeping company in the country, who were famous for the distinctive honey packs sold in most grocery stores. Percy Berry had been instrumental in the freeing up of exports of New Zealand honey, and his two sons were now running the show. Arataki had always sold manuka honey, but now they found it was worth a lot more. And there was Airborne Honey, owned

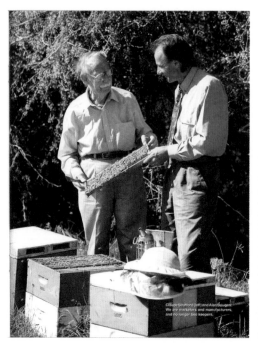

In the 1970s Claude Stratford and Alan Bougen started Comvita in the tiny village of Paengaroa in the Bay of Plenty. The company has been instrumental in the development of manuka honey as a therapeutic product and is now listed on the New Zealand stock exchange, with branches in a number of countries around the world.

by the Bray Family in the South Island, the longest-established honey company in New Zealand. Airborne was a pioneer in the development of 500-gram retail packs of specific floral source honeys, put into in clear plastic PET jars with beautiful, full-colour labels of the flowers themselves. Since they featured all of the country's unique native honeys, manuka was part of their line-up, and it began to attract attention overseas.

Along with these established brands, however, several other companies appeared that were new to the beekeeping scene. The most successful of these was Comvita, a business that started in the 1970s as a health-food store with mail order in the tiny village of Paengaroa in the rural Bay of Plenty. The founder, Claude Stratford, had a long and chequered career in a variety of professions, and was a longtime beekeeper, although not of any great size. However, when he teamed up with the energetic Alan Bougen — a young man imbued with ideas taken from the worldwide movement we might loosely call the 'counter-culture' — bee products became the major focus of the company.* Alan had developed an interest in honey bees when he lived for a time on Great Barrier Island, and in fact it was Les Blackwell who gave him some of his first beekeeping lessons. Claude, on the other hand, was keen on bee products because of their therapeutic properties, and he famously took a teaspoon of bee pollen every day of his very long life. (He lived just shy of his 103rd birthday, and worked six and a half days a week until he was 95.) When the special antibacterial activity of manuka honey was discovered it was a perfect fit, and Comvita eventually grew into the largest bee-products company in Australasia by promoting the medicinal properties of manuka honey. For the first time in modern history, a honey was being marketed to the public specifically for something other than its being good to eat.

Bill Floyd's bald patch and the birth of UMF™

A day before Bill Floyd faxed the famous manuka honey press release, an item appeared on the main evening news broadcast in New Zealand. It featured a man named Reg Day, who was suffering from a terrible leg ulcer that just wouldn't heal, and his family doctor, who had managed to find a cure. The doctor had not used the standard regimen of antibiotics and pressure bandages, however. Instead, he had applied honey straight out of the bottle ... manuka honey to be exact. The segment, presented by the much-loved newsreader Judy Bailey, also included an interview with Peter Molan, in which he said that, even at 50 times dilution, high-activity manuka honey could completely stop the growth of bacteria. For his part, Reg's doctor simply said the honey gave excellent results.*

Alan Bougen remembers that it was after the Reg Day story appeared on TV that sales of Comvita manuka honey in New Zealand really started to grow. And it was Bill Floyd, once again, who managed to get the media interested in the Reg Day case.

As we have seen, at the same time further research was also being conducted into the special, non-peroxide antibacterial activities of manuka honey. Varieties of honeys were being tested at Waikato University against the seven

UNIQUE MANUKA FACTOR'
HONEY ASSOCIATION

The logo of the Unique Manuka Factor Honey Association, holders of the UMF trademark.

most common species of bacteria found in wound infections. All were effective, even when diluted. However, manuka honey with an average level of non-peroxide activity was found to be effective against *Staphylococcus aureus*, even when diluted down with water to a concentration of only 1.8%. By a wide margin, this potentially dangerous bacterial species was most sensitive to manuka. Species of skin fungi that caused athletes' foot were also killed by the honey.*

Peter himself then published a paper detailing the work done at Waikato Hospital that showed that strains of methicillin-resistant *S. aureus* (MRSA) were completely inhibited at 10% honey concentration, a finding that was later confirmed by Rose Cooper, who had begun undertaking pioneering research of her own on manuka honey in Wales.* Peter's university lab was also being inundated with samples of the honey from beekeepers, and a service was being offered to test them for their activity, employing the same method that Kerry Simpson and Peter had first used back in 1988. Results were expressed as a comparison with those dilutions of phenol, and honey marketers began using the percentage figures on their labels. Eventually the demand was so strong that it was given over to certified commercial laboratories.

Both the research and the publicity were starting to make a real difference to the fortunes of the product. According to the July 1995 issue of *The New Zealand Beekeeper* magazine, 'The commercial value of manuka honey doubled in two years.' And Bill Bracks, who later became board chairman of Comvita, remembers doing a 'pencil forecast in 1991 on one page of paper' outlining possible sales growth for the company. 'You needed something to aim for,' says Bill, but the figures looked 'way over the top. We were a $1.2 million a year company, and I was predicting sales in the order of $4 million to 5 million in five years.' In the end they reached their target in just over half that time.*

But then, in 1998, the New Zealand Ministry of Health clamped down on any retail packs of manuka honey that made reference to its antibacterial activity, even if batch samples of the honey had been tested at a recognised laboratory. Both Peter Molan and Bill Floyd remember making the trip to Wellington to argue the case on behalf of the beekeeping industry with ministry officials. Peter had brought with him a large pile of advertising circulars for household cleansers, soaps and mouthwashes; all of them made a similar statement about the product being 'antibacterial'.

At lunchtime they recall going outside to eat their sandwiches and think the problem over. The ministry wouldn't budge: under the Food Act you couldn't make claims about products, and honey was clearly listed there as a food. It was a sunny day in Wellington, and Bill wasn't wearing a hat. Being a redhead, and also not having all that much hair (beard not withstanding), he began feeling a light tingling on his bald patch as the strong New Zealand sun began to burn. Then it occurred to him: couldn't they use some sort of an acronym, like the SPF ratings on sunscreens? They tossed the idea around a bit further. The antibacterial activity Peter and Kerry Simpson had discovered was different from that of other honeys because it wasn't caused by hydrogen peroxide. It was, in fact, 'unique'. And thus was born the idea of using 'UMF' for 'unique manuka factor', three letters that eventually became a brand, registered as a trademark by a group of beekeepers and honey marketers who decided to work co-operatively to enhance the reputation of manuka honey.*

Very early on they saw the need to put some guarantees in place around the use of the gel-diffusion assay tests, the phenol-equivalence ratings, and the statements made to consumers about the strength of the product they were buying. Their foresight led to the creation of this quality mark, audited in the marketplace, which can only be used by the association's members.

Getting a gong

The Queen's Honours List is a special tradition in many of the countries that were formerly part of the British Empire. While it has a lot of the pomp and circumstance associated with its medieval origins (which would involve, as it still sometimes does, the famous tapping on the shoulders with a sword), it is a way for those countries to recognise the dedicated work of people in the community, especially when they have had an important impact on the lives of others. In New Zealand, everybody checks out the list when it appears in the newspapers twice a year, on New Year's Eve and Queen's Birthday. It's a small country, with a famously small number of degrees of separation, and it's usually the case that you know someone getting one of the various medals that people often call a 'gong'.

That was certainly how it was for beekeepers on Queen's Birthday Weekend (not her real birthday, just a public holiday) in June 1995, when Peter Molan, recently promoted to associate professor at the University of Waikato, was awarded an MBE (Member of the British Empire). The government is responsible for deciding who is honoured, based on submissions from the public, organisations and institutions, and they had recognised his pioneering research into the antibacterial attributes of manuka honey. The citation read: 'His work has been the single most important factor in both the domestic and international change in perspective regarding the value of New Zealand honeys.'

A gong is something that is normally awarded to honour a lifetime's achievement. In the case of Peter Molan, however, much of his work in popularising his research on manuka honey, as well as his help in developing its use in woundcare, had only just begun. Peter was still lecturing university students, as well as continuing with research work on various facets of honey, both on his own account and through the projects of his graduate students. But, beyond that, he kept up an amazing pace publicising those research results. Throughout his career, Peter has been an object lesson to every scientist that the job is only half done if you can't explain your results using plain language in a way the rest of the world can understand.

More than anything, he has an enormous enthusiasm for his subject. It comes out in his writing, and of course far more in the many talks he has given all around the world. If you are in the audience you can't help but be caught up by it all. He is fascinated by this substance which he once knew absolutely nothing about; how the bees make it, how wonderfully self-preserving it is, how strongly it can deal to potentially life-threatening bacteria, and what an almost perfect wound dressing it makes. The more Peter has studied it, the more amazing things it has revealed. It is a simple substance which most of us just take for granted, but which is turning out to be so much more. Just as he took apart his parents' clock when he was a child, he and his fellow scientists have been figuring out more and more about how honey works. And he can't help but share that sense of discovery with the world.

'Snatching defeat from the jaws of victory'

Beekeepers are a very small minority, both in New Zealand and worldwide. In New Zealand there are only 500 or so owners of commercial beekeeping outfits, and probably no more than about 1500 people (owners and employees) who make their living full-time by keeping bees. Worldwide it's much the same. There are about 72 million beehives, but no statistics exist on how many people keep them on a commercial basis. If we use a ratio similar to New Zealand's as comparison, however, that equates to probably no more than 270,000 people making their livelihoods from beekeeping. That's 0.0038% of the total population of the planet.

There are, of course, many more people who keep bees as a hobby. Some take it very seriously, and often put considerable effort and expenditure into what for them is a craft. There are times when they even decide to take the plunge, building up their hive numbers until they give up their 'day job' and try to make a fulltime living from their bees. Others are really just 'bee-havers'. They have a beehive or two in the backyard, or on a friend's farm, but don't manage the bees on anything like a regular basis. They might harvest some honey on the odd occasion, but often the bees become so neglected that they eventually either starve or die from a disease like varroa, the parasitic mite that, if left untreated, will eventually kill any honey bee colony.

Most beekeepers in the world are hobbyists, and even if all the hives they maintain are taken into account, they do not contribute that many bee colonies to the environment – certainly nowhere near the number needed to pollinate the commercially produced food we eat. It is the other group, the commercial operators, who manage the vast number of beehives that are so important to us all. Commercial beekeepers are well aware that they are part of a tiny minority group, and they are used to being thought of as a little 'peculiar' by their neighbours. In most cases they keep bees because they are truly captivated by them as creatures, and especially by how bees manage to produce something of value to humans almost (as it were) out of thin air.

The lawyer and former New Zealand politician Stephen Franks, who has chaired meetings of commercial beekeepers, believes they're a different breed. 'They're not a normal sample of the population,' he reckons. 'They're intelligent, curious, reflective. They believe in the moral goodness of what they do. They're self-reliant and opinionated. And they think if you disagree with them then you're against them and you're a bad person.'* There's certainly a lot of truth in that, because as we have seen, it takes a 'different' sort of person to spend most days cooped up in a set of overalls and veil, never quite being able to put out of their mind the potentially painful stings of their charges. And of course commercial beekeepers are always competitive, and sometimes aggressively so. They often hold long-standing grudges over apiary sites, and sometimes even honey sales, in a way that is almost incomprehensible to dairy farmers or kiwifruit growers. They are also invariably 'self-made', unless they have taken over the business from their parents. It doesn't take any land or even extensive capital to go beekeeping. You can build up a business, beehive by beehive, investing the proceeds from one to pay for another, and by splitting the actual colonies of bees you can easily make more of the same.

Producing honey is also very dependent on the weather, probably more so than for any other agricultural industry. You can do everything right — keep the bees healthy, well fed, with plenty of room so they don't swarm and have somewhere to store the honey crop. But it all comes down to a very short period (often just three weeks) in late spring or early summer. If it rains too much, or the weather is too cold for the plants to secrete lots of nectar, you don't get a crop. So as you can imagine, that sort of pressure isn't always highly conducive to maintaining a positive attitude to life.

Commercial beekeepers usually have intricate relationships with each other. On the one hand they need someone to share their passion with (and almost without exception beekeepers decide to become commercial because of their obsession, not out of any sense of being able to get rich quick). On the other hand, they generally need to hold at least some things close to their chest, lest their mates steal a march on them. It is an agricultural occupation, and yet one that is a true breeding ground for entrepreneurialism. This is at least part of the reason why there is also tension when it comes to their associations and industry affairs.

All this is by way of some sort of explanation for what happened to the planning efforts of the National Beekeepers' Association through to the end of the 1990s, and particularly the efforts of Bill Floyd in helping develop the profile of New Zealand honey. Just a year after having approved the hive levy that put Bill to work on their honey marketing plan, the National Beekeepers' Association executive decided to reduce the levy per hive for marketing to 30 cents, decreasing the plan's $150,000 budget by 40%. It took a special meeting forced by the membership to increase the levy again by 5 cents.

In the years that followed, the money being spent on marketing was a significant source of discussion at the annual conferences of the association. Some argued that the increased levy needed to pay for the work would drive beekeepers underground, since the system relied on an honest declaration of hive numbers to make it all work. Others said things like, 'The tree has just been planted, let's not pull it out of the ground', and 'We seem to be trying to snatch defeat from the jaws of victory'. Eventually the programme was wound back to the point where Bill Floyd was left with no choice but to resign. Priorities had changed in the New Zealand beekeeping industry, and beekeepers were being faced with the most serious threat ever posed to their livelihoods: the discovery of the dreaded varroa parasite in Auckland in 2000.

Bill went on to work with a number of other New Zealand food sectors, including the famous green-lipped mussels and salmon industries. These days he manages the International Blackcurrant Association, and uses many of the techniques he learned during his time with honey to help people better understand the health-giving properties of that fruit.

'I often think back and wish I was still working with the New Zealand honey industry,' he says. ' "Iconic" is such an abused word these days, but its definition is "a magnet of positive meaning", and I think that, in that respect, New Zealand honeys really are iconic of its regions and the country as a whole. In all my travels, I don't think I have been to a country that has such a wonderful expression of different honeys. And we have got a number of sources of honey that come from native plants that don't really exist anywhere else in the world. As for manuka, it has become the star of the show.'*

A honey fit for a queen

The tension between co-operative endeavour and rugged individualism became too much for the marketing plans of the National Beekeepers' Association. But in the end it really didn't matter. As Bill Floyd says, 'What I have learned in life is that marketing budgets can speed up the rate of success, but you still have to have the right idea.' And the entrepreneurial zeal of a number of New Zealanders was taking manuka honey, and the work of Peter Molan and others, to countries and cultures as diverse as Australia, China, the United Kingdom and Japan.

Comvita is now listed on the New Zealand stock exchange, and is probably one of the few bee-products companies in the world to have ever achieved that feat. It has grown over 20 times in turnover compared with the figure Bill Bracks once pencilled in on his handmade spreadsheet, and is now arguably the biggest therapeutic bee-products company in the world. Others, like Manuka Health and Manukamed, have come on-stream, while established players like Arataki and Airborne are also doing well.

The value of honey exports from New Zealand grew at a compound rate of 30% between 2000 and 2010, and the country receives a dramatically higher average price for its honeys than its competitors in the international marketplace. A big reason for this is manuka, which is now worth over $140 million per year. It is being used as a food ingredient because of its unique flavour, in cosmetics, as a natural health product, and as a mainstream medical treatment.*

Beekeepers are moving their bees out of the pasture apiaries they once used to produce clover honey, as well as giving away lucrative kiwifruit pollination contracts, to get as close to the big areas of manuka scrub as they can. And hive numbers have sky-rocketed. There are now 150,000 more hives in the country than there were when varroa first struck in 2000, an increase of 50%.*

In the beekeeping outfit that I once helped run in Northland, we managed to place all of our apiaries throughout hundreds of square kilometres of territory without any of them (well, at least almost any of them) being close enough to stands of manuka to 'contaminate' the honey crop. Twenty years later, when you look at a map of hive locations in the district it is as if that outfit now exists in a kind of parallel universe. In that same overall area, the apiaries have been put in completely different locations, as close as possible to the bush and scrub that produce copious quantities of manuka honey. Because the timing of commercial pollination interferes with this early-season honey production, a business run by a different beekeeper now provides that service to growers. And demand for both the honey, as well as choice locations on which to site hives, has resulted in at least one case of 'bee rustling', with a local man convicted of stealing hives. It is the same right throughout the country.

New Zealand honey has always been precious, from the time Mary Bumby first offered it at the mission station in Mangungu, to when Les Blackwell's grandfather provided pohutukawa honey for King George V. But in 2011 it was the turn of the New Zealand prime minister to give honey as a royal gift. The honey he took to Windsor Castle as a luncheon present was a Kiwi product people all around the world were now talking about. It was manuka honey, and nothing could speak more loudly about the change to its fortunes than that it was now seen as 'fit for a Queen'.*

Five

MERELY
A WEED

Geographically speaking, there are actually two East Capes in New Zealand. The first is a bumpy point, right at the end of the big, horn-shaped chunk of land that juts out into the Pacific halfway down the east coast of the North Island. Locals say it's the first place in the world to see the sun each day, due to its easternmost position in the country, and the decision by a world conference in 1884 to draw the international date-line many hundreds of kilometres out in the ocean further east. That claim is hotly disputed, though, not just by an offshore part of New Zealand called the Chatham Islands. Samoa now also lays claims to the title, having decided to jump time zones in 2011. In so doing, it put itself on the western side of that imaginary but essential starting boundary that marks the beginning of each day (although in the process the people of Samoa paid for privilege by losing a full 24 hours they couldn't get back).

The East Cape isn't just a point of land that sees an early sunrise, however. It is also an entire region of the country. And like many similar areas of New Zealand, it is hard to know just where the East Cape begins and ends. Many, in fact, would say 'The Cape' is more than anything a special state of mind. It is certainly one of the remoter places on the North Island, and is famous for its laidback lifestyle, rugged coastline, and steep hills leading back up into the dense rainforest that is the Ureweras.

It may be remote, but every Kiwi school child knows that the southernmost reach of the East Cape region was the first piece of New Zealand sighted by Captain Cook, when in 1769 he made his voyage of discovery aboard the *Endeavour*. Or rather, it was the 12-year-old surgeon's boy, Nicholas Young, who saw gleaming white cliffs at the southernmost end of a bay, and was rewarded with both the naming of that point (Young Nick's Head), and a gallon of rum. Unfortunately, however, that location, which in generations to come became the district's main centre of population (Gisborne) and an area of bountiful horticulture, was branded 'Poverty Bay' by the normally positively-disposed Cook, because, as he said, 'It afforded us no one thing we wanted'. This was supposedly in reference to his crew not being able to obtain the wood, water and fresh food they needed, not (so it is said) their getting off on the wrong foot with local Maori.

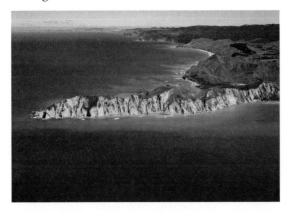

Young Nick's Head, near Gisborne, the gleaming white cliffs first seen by Nicholas Young, the surgeon's boy on the *Endeavour*, on 7 October 1769.

Whatever the name, agricultural development in the region certainly changed the native plant-covered flats and hills into sheep and cattle country. After World War II, more difficult pieces of land were brought into production, with farmers receiving grants from the government to knock down native scrub and sow the resulting bare ground with grass. The ground itself, however, was unstable, particularly on steep slopes, and when the East Cape faced the fury of a terrible cyclone called Bola in 1988, hillsides slumped into valleys and streams throughout the region. Many farms were scenes of devastation, and people began to reassess the viability of pasture-based agriculture in some locations. As a result, the growing of the exotic species *Pinus radiata* for timber, which was already an important part of the New Zealand economy, took on more prominence in the East Cape, especially since the roots of the trees were able to help stabilise erosion-prone land.

And so it was in November 1992 — almost a year to the day after Bill Floyd had faxed his famous press release — that the Minister of Agriculture was interviewed on *Rural Report*, a nationwide radio programme listened to by many of the nation's farmers, about a new project for the East Cape that had recently been announced by the government. The scheme would involve the planting of some 200,000 hectares of *Pinus radiata*, using substantial government subsidies. The hope was that it would help control erosion in the region brought on by the cyclone, and also provide new economic opportunities.

Unfortunately, however, the project was designed to do a lot more than just plant up eroded areas of the Cape. It was also going to clear for forestry up to 75,000 hectares of manuka and kanuka. These two native species had always grown on the steep slopes of the East Cape and kept the hillsides in place, but ironically they had been cut down in their millions over previous decades to bring into production much of the land that was now being seen as needing erosion control. But not all of those native 'shrubs' to be destroyed in the government's new scheme were the product of recent regeneration. Some of the stands of manuka and kanuka destined for the chop were said to contain amazing old-growth specimens up to five storeys high and wider across than an oil drum.*

Local beekeepers attended a public meeting on the issue in Gisborne, and Peter Molan was asked to come to the city early the next year to speak on his research into manuka honey. But the government didn't seem particularly fazed. In the *Rural Report* interview, the Minister, whose name was John Falloon, replied to a question on the subject by simply saying, 'I mean, after all, manuka is merely a weed'.*

The ubiquitous shrub

Unfortunately the plight of manuka on the East Cape isn't all that unique. In fact, it is just another chapter in the long and very chequered history of what is by most botanists' reckoning the most widely spread and populous of New Zealand's native trees and shrubs. You come across it wherever you go in the country, from just below Cape Reinga at the tip of the North Island, all the way down to Bluff at the bottom end of the South Island. And as we saw in our brief excursion to Great Barrier, it is quite at home on many of the various coastal islands as well.

You won't find many manuka plants as big as those giants destined to be cut down on the Cape. Nevertheless, they can take on an amazing variety of shapes and sizes, from a small shrub that almost lies along the ground, to something resembling a small tree, at 4 to 8 metres high.*

Manuka clings to coastal headlands, bending its many-branched tops into the gales, and manages to survive even when being routinely covered with salt-spray. It climbs high up the sides of mountains to positions that would normally be considered above the tree-line. And it doesn't care whether it has the very best sort of land, or takes up residence in poor to almost non-existent soil. In fact, manuka has even figured out how to stay alive with its roots more or less permanently in water. In lake-side and swampy situations, manuka can create specialised ventilating tissue called *aerenchyma*, which are air channels in the leaves, stems and roots of some plants that allow the exchange of gases between the shoots and the root. The tissues are a bit like internal snorkels, and help manuka plants to live on with their roots fully submerged.*

Under some circumstances, where the bigger, slower-growing species of the native forest find it hard going, manuka can form permanent stands. But because it produces so much seed, grows so fast, and loves the light, manuka is also one of nature's great restorers. It's a 'pioneer' (or *seral*) species that springs up after some sort of disturbance has destroyed the often great and slower-growing trees in the native forest, whether they be the massive kauri in the northern parts of the North Island, the podocarps like totara, or those beech forests that in some of the northern parts of the South Island produce the honeydew collected by honey bees. Manuka keeps the soil from eroding, and by adding leaf matter, prepares the ground for the regeneration process that eventually, through a series of succession species (called *seral communities*), results in the climax forest establishing itself once again.

But being 'beneficial' to others isn't necessarily the main thing that most plants are about. In point of fact, manuka would probably like to take over the whole of both islands, if it could just figure out how to eliminate all those climax forest species, and then keep the forest from re-growing. It is just so well-suited to the place. As it is, it has to be content with situations that the forest doesn't like, as well as setting up shop as one of the first species after fires and other, often human, disruptions, only to eventually be muscled out (sometimes up to a century later) by the juvenile forms of the forest giants.

In fact, it is this fundamental drive that all organisms have to make as many copies of themselves as they can that has created problems for manuka. If it just grew more slowly, and hid in the dark recesses of the bush, it probably would never have become such an issue in the agricultural development of the country. But it just can't help itself. When a farmer clears some land, particularly in the hill country, but doesn't graze it intensely, manuka is very likely to 'jump the fence'. As we will see, that love for newly opened spaces does much to explain why even in 1992 it wasn't just the Minister of Agriculture who thought manuka was a weed.

Phar Lap and the fly-paper of the Pacific

Before we go much further, we need to deal with something that is likely to cause a fair bit of consternation, particularly if you happen to be a dyed-in-the-wool New Zealander. Kiwis, and their Aussie mates across the Tasman, like nothing better than to engage in friendly banter. And apart from successes or otherwise on the sports field, one of the major topics of discussion is which country can rightly claim ownership to various icons known around the world. For instance, Australians pretend that Phar Lap, one of the most famous racehorses that ever lived, was theirs. As New Zealanders point out, however, this thoroughbred with an enormous heart (literally, since it was twice normal size) was born and bred in the South Island.

So what of manuka, the plant that produces a honey now known throughout the world? It has a name given to it by Maori, and almost all manuka honey is made in New Zealand. It is a real Kiwi icon, so surely it has always been part of the place since the time it set off from Gondwanaland? Right? Well, actually wrong. Scientists have now come to the view that rather than New Zealand being the famous 'Moa's Ark' we mentioned in a previous chapter, it may in fact have been the 'Fly-Paper of the Pacific'.*

That's perhaps an unfortunate term for something that seems quite reasonable, given that the country consists of two very big islands that, while physically separated from the rest of the world for 80 million years, have always been lapped by waters that could carry seeds and spores, as well as being a very large perch for birds flying across the sea. And it goes both ways: New Zealand has at times also contributed plants in the other direction.

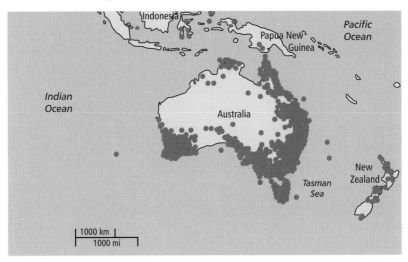

The natural range for most *Leptospermum* species is restricted to Australasia, but several have managed to establish in south-east Asia.

The movements we are talking about are rare occurrences, but given the vast amount of time involved, it takes only a very few seeds of the right species, with a real liking for a particular niche, for that plant to grow into abundance. And that is what DNA analysis — the amazing technique that is unlocking the way living things have changed over time — has shown us. Many species we take for granted as being 'originals' in fact arrived in New Zealand a lot later on. Far fewer appear to have been residents for that entire span of time. But we hardly need DNA tests to discover where manuka originally came from. We can work that out on our own. Manuka is in the *Leptospermum* genus (*letpo* = small or slender; *spermum* = seed), and by latest count there are a total of 88 *Leptospermum* species in the world, all with the distinctive seed capsules (the dried 'fruits') containing many fine seeds.* For anyone thinking manuka was somehow unique to New Zealand, however, the bad news is that 86 of those species are also found in Australia, while two more have managed to make their way to South East Asia, one sitting on Mt Kinabalu in Borneo, and the other sticking to the mountains in Myanmar, Thailand, the Philippines, and various Indonesian islands.

Now species being what they are, and taking a very long time to separate themselves enough from their relatives so that they can't generally mate with them and successfully produce lots of viable offspring, it is almost inevitable that manuka came from overseas. Otherwise there would most probably be a lot more *Leptospermum* species on Moa's Ark, with their seed capsules making their way to the surf, and a lot fewer across the Tasman Sea.

Manuka, known to the botanists as *Leptospermum scoparium* (*scoparium* = a broom), may be the only *Leptospermum* species present as a native plant in New Zealand, but if you were concentrating on the maths two paragraphs ago, you will already have guessed that it is also found in Australia. *L. scoparium* isn't widely distributed on that country's mainland, however, being found only on the southern coast of New South Wales down to western Victoria. It is more prevalent in Tasmania, though, an island with a climate much more similar to that of the South Island of New Zealand. And if any further evidence is needed, it turns out manuka is the only New Zealand species that releases its seeds during a fire, something which of course is very common with a wide range of Australian native plants.*

But while the origin of manuka might be the sort of thing Aussies love to needle Kiwis about, as is often the case it is the New Zealanders who are able to have the last laugh. While *Leptospermum scoparium* might be an immigrant, it nevertheless has found that it loves almost every environmental condition the varied climate and geography of New Zealand can throw at it. The only thing it can't seem to handle is the extreme harshness of the Australian Outback.

Manuka and kanuka get a helping hand

Joy Thompson, from the Royal Botanic Gardens in Sydney, has written the definitive compendium on the *Leptospermum* genus. She says all the evidence points to the parent of all those species having originated in Australia before that continent became arid in what is called the middle Miocene period (from 15 to 11 million years ago).* The change to a much harsher climate then isolated the parent into a number of separate pockets, and it needed to adapt to dwindling resources and the increased frequency of fires. So it was the pressures of natural selection that created all the many species.

The one that would eventually be called manuka, however, arrived on New Zealand's shores well after that time. No one knows for sure when or how, but *Leptospermum scoparium* certainly isn't one of the more ancient forms. At the same time, though, it is not so far removed from its many Australian relatives that it can't be crossed successfully with at least some of them.

A lot less is known about kanuka, currently identified botanically as *Kunzea ericoides* (*Kunzea* = the Latin form for Kunze, the name of the German naturalist who discovered it; *ericoides* = similar to *Erica*, the heathers and heaths). In fact, it wasn't until the ever-precise Joy Thompson put kanuka in the *Kunzea* genus in 1983 that it was thought to be anything other than a *Leptospermum*.

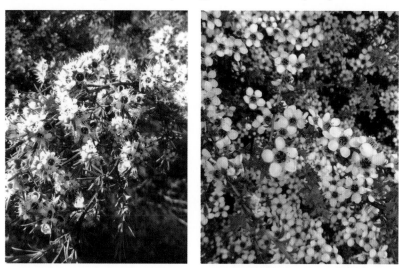

Kanuka (*Kunzea ericoides*) is often confused with manuka. The leaves of kanuka (left) are softer and the branches often look feathery, while the flowers of manuka (right) are larger.

Regardless of the names botanists give them, however, kanuka and manuka are certainly closely related. The casual observer often has a difficult time telling them apart (the leaves of kanuka are softer and the branches often look feathery, while the flowers of manuka are larger). And a non-fertile cross between kanuka and manuka found on Great Barrier Island (which another botanist maintains is a separate species), shows that the two may not be all that distant from each other after all.*

Kanuka and manuka are sometimes found living together, although kanuka is better able to handle the driest conditions of environments like Central Otago. On the other hand, it isn't able to make those internal snorkels like manuka can, so kanuka won't stand wet feet. And it can't handle the low-fertility soils or higher elevations that manuka has made its own. Kanuka does grow taller, however, and in fact those monsters that were scheduled to be cut down on the East Cape might even have been misidentified as their usually smaller relatives. Some kanuka up to 20 metres high and over 200 years old have been found. Finally, as any beekeeper will tell you, kanuka blooms later than manuka, although, as we will see, if you go by the colour of flowers you can sometimes be fooled.

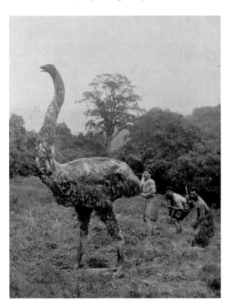

The pursuit of giant moa by Maori when they first came to New Zealand opened up much of the country to the spread of manuka and kanuka. This depiction of a mock hunt was produced for the 1906–7 Christchurch International Exhibition.

What is fairly certain, however, is that manuka and kanuka weren't all that widely distributed throughout the North and South Island before the arrival of man. A baseline study of what the New Zealand environment was like in 3000 BC — before both the cataclysm of the Taupo eruption in the central North Island about 1800 years ago, and first records of Polynesian settlement some thousand years later — shows that 85–90% of the country was covered in forest.* There were plenty of bogs, and riverbeds prone to flooding, though, as well as steep cliffs and volcanic rock, and studies of pollen found in soil and sediment samples show that manuka and kanuka had managed to find a home in some of these non-forested places. But their breakout to so much more of the environment needed help, and they got it in the form of the Maori, who were the first humans to significantly alter what was the last major settled landmass on Earth.

It may come as something of a surprise to many modern-day New Zealanders, but the spread of manuka and kanuka throughout much of New Zealand had everything to do with the actions of humans, rather than simply nature itself. In their search for that major source of protein — the giant flightless bird they called the moa — Maori began to set fire to parts of the forest. This, in turn, encouraged the bursting of the seed pods of the manuka and kanuka in areas now clear enough for them to establish themselves. Nonetheless, this opportunity to spread their growing locations was time-sensitive, for while *middens* (the piles of kitchen waste that archaeologists find so illuminating) at first mostly contained bird and marine mammal bones, 300 years later the middens contained mainly shellfish remains. Moa were no longer a major source of food, and of course they finally became extinct.

The sudden change creating major non-forested areas had been completed by about 1600, and, by the time Mary Bumby brought those first honey bees to Mangungu in 1839, about half of the original forest that covered New Zealand was no longer there. By that time, manuka and kanuka had well and truly jumped in to take the missing forest's place.

A Maori pharmacy

As manuka and kanuka started spreading themselves around the newly opened-up landscape, Maori found both plants could be very useful for a whole range of things. You could not make massive canoes from their wood like you could with the giant totara, but the long, stout trunks of manuka and kanuka were good for the paddles used to propel the boats through the waves. Manuka sticks were also put on the bottom of canoes as something a bit dry for the paddlers to sit and kneel on.

The wood was also valued for the manufacture of a range of implements because it was so hard and strong. Of particular importance was its use in the making of *korere*, sacred vessels and funnels used to feed chiefs at times of high *tapu* (spiritual restriction), when they were not allowed to touch food and therefore had to be fed.* Other, more domestic implements included bowls, fernroot beaters, mauls, garden cultivators (*ketu*), digging sticks (*ko*) and hoes (*hoto*). And manuka poles also came in handy when hunting, as a spear for both fish and birds, and in the making of eel-pots. They also made excellent handles for scoop-nets. The long, straight trees were sometimes used in the construction of storage platforms, and the bark was a very durable roofing material, although totara was preferred.

Presaging what Peter Molan would discover much later in manuka honey (a product which of course didn't exist before about 1840), Maori also found that the plant itself was a veritable pharmacy. It was especially useful when an infusion made from its leaves was taken to treat urinary tract infections. According to one overly Victorian commentator, the potion was 'peculiarly serviceable to persons in a reduced state whose previous moralities would not admit of the strictest investigation'. A tea made from manuka leaves was also a remedy for diarrhoea and dysentery, while inhaling the steaming vapours relieved the symptoms of cold. A drink made by boiling manuka's inner bark was said to reduce fever, and, when cold, the same liquid served as a gargle and mouthwash. The outer bark was helpful for mouth, throat and eye troubles. Even the seed pods were put to good use. They were given to babies to chew for colic, with 6–8 berries given every 10 minutes until the pain decreased. And a poultice made by pounding the seed pods was applied to wounds or running sores.

While manuka honey may not have been available until the arrival of the English, the plant did provide one sweet treat for Maori. A sugary resin was sometimes found on the young branches of manuka in summer, probably caused by insect damage, and this gum (called *pia* or *tohika*) was sought after by both children and adults. It was also something of a salve for burns, provided a lozenge for coughs, and was given to babies to ease constipation.

Manuka is a name that pretty much the whole world knows now, almost entirely because of the honey that bees produce from its flowers. But of course it is a Maori word, since those amazing Polynesian seafarers, who travelled the South Pacific Ocean 400 years before any Europeans, were the first humans to encounter the plant in the new land they called Aotearoa. As you would imagine, however, given that the shrub was so widespread and useful, they didn't just have one term for it. Six more besides manuka are recorded in modern *te reo* dictionaries, including *kahikatoa, katoa, pata, rauwiri, rauiri* and *tara manuka*. This last describes the belief some tribes had that manuka was the female tree, whereas kanuka (or *toa manuka*) was the male. Just like modern New Zealanders, however, Maori didn't necessarily always distinguish between the two species, sometimes using the same words for both. Other differentiating names for kanuka, however, included *kopuka, manuka-rauriki, manuea* and *maru*. *Kahikatoa* is still used by some Maori in the northernmost parts of New Zealand, and there is a theory that it means 'weapon', whereas manuka and kanuka are the two types of plant used for that purpose.* This might be similar to the way the English use one name for both a punishment stick and a type of tree, as in 'the headmaster gave me the birch'.

Captain James Cook, award-winning brewer

During the Age of Discovery it didn't take the Europeans long to start naming all the new plants and animals they encountered in what was for them, at least, the various 'new' parts of the world. The Enlightenment's penchant for systematic inquisitiveness resulted in Linnaeus starting to categorise all living things. And as new plants — either alive or as preserved samples — were brought back to Europe and deposited into private collections and museums, the categorisers (called *taxonomists*) assigned them descriptive Latin and sometimes Greek words – one for the grouping of close relations (the *genus*), and the other for the *species* itself.

We have already met briefly one of the most famous of those plant-discovery expeditions, at the beginning of this chapter. When Young Nick spied the white cliffs at the southern end of the East Cape in 1769, on board the *Endeavour* with Captain Cook was the greatest botanist of his time, Joseph Banks, together with his self-financed entourage of nine servants and artists. Banks would eventually return to England with the pressed leaves and flowers of over 30,000 plants. In so doing he increased the number of species in the world recorded by European taxonomists by fully one quarter.*

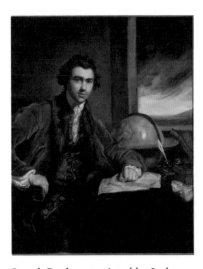

Joseph Banks, as painted by Joshua Reynolds. Banks and his assistant Daniel Solander collected the first samples of manuka the very first day they set foot on New Zealand soil, but later mis-identified the plant as a *Philadelphus* (mock-orange).

With their record as great collectors, it probably comes as no surprise that Banks and his fellow botanist Daniel Solander secured a sample of manuka. And if the date is correct on the remarkably well-preserved, mounted specimen now held at Te Papa, the National Museum of New Zealand, they did so along the shores of the soon-to-be-named Poverty Bay on the very first day that anyone from Britain ever set foot on New Zealand soil.*

When you look up *Leptospermum scoparium* in the botany books, however, you won't find the names 'Banks and Solander' attached at the end, even though there are whole genera commemorating them, like the Australian shrubs *Banksia*, and species names like *solanderi* and variations (including that *Nothofagus* species we looked at previously, N. *solandri,* that produces New Zealand honeydew). The reason is that Banks and Solander didn't officially name it, at least so far as taxonomists were concerned.

Along the east coast of the North Island, the *Endeavour* dropped the botanists ashore further north on the East Cape, at Mercury Bay along the Coromandel Peninsula, and in the Bay of Islands, as well as on the northernmost tip of the South Island. In all they collected 350 new plants, which they described in botanical detail in a manuscript. But unfortunately the book was never published. This is probably just as well, however, since Solander, for all his great skill in plant classification, incorrectly described both manuka and kanuka as being in the genus *Philadelphus* (mock-orange).*

The honour of naming rights went instead to J.R. Forster and his son George, who accompanied Cook on his second voyage to New Zealand, aboard the *Resolution*. The Forsters collected samples of manuka at that same tip of the South Island, in Queen Charlotte Sound, and their names were attached to the Latin genus and species they gave it in published form upon their return to England in 1776.*

Naming rights or not, Captain Cook and his crew immediately found several practical uses for manuka. Like the Maori, they used its leaves to brew a tea, and it became so popular later on that settlers, both in New Zealand and Australia, gave it the common name 'tea tree'. The problem with common names, however, is that they often aren't that discerning, which helps explain why the Australians also use the name 'tea tree' or 'ti tree' to refer to a completely different genus of native plant known scientifically as *Melaleuca*.

On Cook's second voyage, when the *Resolution* anchored in the darkly primeval confines of Dusky Sound on the far southwest coast of the South Island, the crew also used manuka leaves to make a rather more potent drink, becoming the first persons to brew beer in New Zealand. In addition to manuka, they used the droopy leaves of the rimu, a tall and stately conifer that would go on to provide essential building timbers for generations of New Zealand houses. The recipe followed one that had earlier been described by Banks in his journals of a voyage along the Newfoundland coast, half a world away. In that concoction they used North American black spruce, and to Cook and his thirsty crew the two local native species must have looked close enough. They boiled the leaves down, strained the liquid, added molasses, then once it had cooled, put it into casks along with a little yeast. To one crew member, at least, it 'bubbled and tasted rather like champagne'. As for Cook, he was so impressed that he later said: 'Had I known better how this beer would have succeeded and the greater use it was to people I would have come better provided.'

While its usefulness to men on a long voyage away from the grog shops of Britain was obvious, it is said that the main reason for Cook allowing beer to be made in Dusky Sound was rather more medicinal. Scurvy was then the dreaded enemy of anyone making a prolonged voyage at sea; if you signed on, you generally had a 50:50 chance of being killed by the disease.

At the time, the Royal Navy was conducting experiments in an attempt to alleviate the problem, and Cook took with him several foodstuffs that it was thought might help. These *antiscorbutics* included 30 gallons of carrot marmalade and 100 pounds of sauerkraut for each person on board. At the same time, however,

Cook made sure the crew had fresh greens and beverages wherever they stopped, and of course brewing was the universally accepted form of *biotechnology* or food transformation used to preserve drinking liquids in a form that wouldn't go off. In any event, Cook's regimes proved amazingly successful. On his first voyage not a single crew member was lost to scurvy, and on completion of the second he was awarded a Royal Society Gold Medal. He was a national hero, and not just for charting the Antipodes.

As some commentators have joked, this first beer brewed in New Zealand was therefore a medal-winning one as well, but of course the recipe didn't really take off in the decades to come. Still, New Zealand boutique breweries have recently begun making a manuka beer, and it doesn't taste half bad.*

'Tickled Pink' and 'Mesmer Eyes'

The other use Europeans immediately put manuka to, along with some of its many *Leptospermum* cousins, was as an ornamental shrub. In less than 10 years after Cook's first voyage, nurseries in England were offering manuka plants for sale to put in your garden, although like Solander they misnamed them as *Philadelphus*.*

While its ability to adapt to a wide range of environments, as well as produce showy displays of flowers, certainly made manuka attractive to horticulturalists, it also had a further attribute — something plant people call *polymorphism*, which in effect means that its great genetic variation appears in the various shapes, sizes and other forms it can take. This is also why it can sometimes be difficult to tell manuka apart from kanuka, and perhaps, as in Solander's case, even mistake manuka for other species of plants. An example is the use of the common names 'red tea tree' and 'white tea tree' for manuka and kanuka. Manuka has a range of flower colours, from pink, to a blush, to bright white. Mutations have also been found, and these have been incorporated into the breeding of remarkable ornamental varieties. The famous pink-flowered manuka variety 'Keatleyi' was found by Captain Keatley at the far northern harbour of Parengarenga, back in 1917, and the amazing red 'Nichollsii' came from a sheep station north of Christchurch in 1898. It made its way to England, and won a major award at the International Horticultural Exhibition at Chelsea in 1912.

Another type of rare mutation in manuka is *double flowers*, where many petals appear, rather than the normal five. A famous white double is 'Leonard Wilson', named after the person who discovered it on Banks Peninsula around 1915–1916. With careful crossings, double-flowering manuka can now often resemble tiny roses.*

Today, manuka is certainly a very important garden plant, leaving its kanuka relative far behind in that respect. In what looks to be a fairly comprehensive list of the creations that plant breeders have registered, a total of 218 cultivars of *Leptospermum* are described, with almost two-thirds identified as related to manuka (*L. scoparium*). The rest are derived from solely Australian species or, in a few cases,

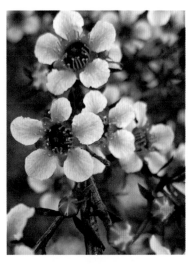

Chance finds of pink and red manuka plants in the wild became the basis for the breeding of many different named varieties for the home garden.

a cross between two species. As always with these things, the names the growers have chosen for their manuka cultivars certainly run the gamut, from the decidedly New Zealand-related ('Weka', 'Tui', 'Kiwi') to the fairly utilitarian ('Weeping Grey', 'Dwarf Form', 'Little Lemon'), as well as the definitely whimsical ('Tickled Pink', 'Rosy Morn', 'Bouffant', and the wonderful 'Mesmer Eyes'). And at least a couple suggest that they might have been given their names after a long, hard, hot day out in the field ('Cherry Brandy', 'Martini' and 'Pink Champagne').

Of the Australian species, favourites for breeding seem to be the natives *Leptospermum polygalifolium*, *L. flavescens*, *L. laevigatum*. Named varieties that are obviously Aussie-inspired include 'Big Red', 'Jervis Bay', 'Shore Tuff', and the hopefully named 'Mozzie Blocker'. That last one may not be as crazy as it seems, however, since *L. petersonii* is grown in commercial plantations in Africa, Central America and Australia because it produces a lemon-scented oil that contains citronellal, a compound found in mosquito-repellent citronella candles.*

And showing how closely related some of these Australia species are, honey collected from *L. polygalifolium*, commonly called jelly bush, has also been found to produce the same special non-peroxide antibacterial activity that has made manuka honey so well known.

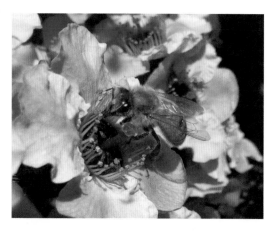

In some limited areas of Australia, bees collect honey with non-peroxide antibacterial activity from the jelly bush (*Leptospermum polygalifolium*).

You will find manuka being grown for its ornamental value literally around the world, from northern Europe, to Israel, South Africa and the United States. It is said to be almost everywhere in Irish gardens, and has even managed to naturalise in Hawaii, where it has escaped from gardens and colonised wet areas. Manuka decorates the streets of San Francisco, forms at least a part of the Lost Gardens of Heligan in Cornwall, and a spectacular specimen adorns Portmeirion, the Potemkin-like village of spectacular eccentricity in northern Wales that was the backdrop for *The Prisoner*, a cult TV series from the 1960s starring Patrick McGoohan. If you know what you are looking for, it is surprising just how often manuka pops up.

Dealing to an 'arch-criminal' weed

In an article in the farming magazine *The New Zealand Journal of Agriculture* in 1967, Jack Fraser, the chairman of the Honey Marketing Authority, argued that 'a major increase in production cannot be expected', and that the future of New Zealand honey marketing lay in the home market. In that regard he particularly mentioned 'more intensive farming methods and land development that have eliminated many native floral resources', and he singled out manuka. While he thought that 'native bush areas could be exploited provided a satisfactory return could be obtained for native honeys on an overseas specialty market', he wasn't hopeful.

Factors given for this conclusion included the fluctuating nature of New Zealand honey production, the introduction of something called *manuka blight*, and the destruction of manuka scrub to develop more farmland.

On the facing page of the article was an advertisement for Caterpillar Tractors that included a picture of a big yellow bulldozer crushing native vegetation, with the headline 'Land Clearing — Key to Higher Profits'. It seems sadly ironic now, but given the general view of manuka at the time, neither the readers nor the editor may have paid it much attention.*

This land-clearing was of course the result of the amazing change that occurred in the New Zealand environment after 1840, a change that turned both the North Island and the South Island into pasture-based agricultural powerhouses, with the result that much of the more accessible land eventually came to resemble a South Pacific version of the English countryside. Maori may have reduced the forest cover by half in their hunt for moa, but Europeans destroyed half of what remained in a shorter period of time.

At the same time, many kinds of plant found their way to the country. Over a 150-year period, on average 11 new plant species per year became established in New Zealand. Some of them were intentionally introduced because of their economic importance, while others came from seeds that one way or another just hitched a ride. Many became noxious weeds, although a number of these (such as gorse) were also extremely well-liked by honey bees. Not all of those weeds were 'exotic', however. Manuka became a scourge to many farmers, both as they began to break in the land, and later. We shouldn't be too harsh on those European settlers in their antipathy towards manuka, however. It was growing literally everywhere, and its density and ability to regenerate in pasture made it a real foe of both light and vistas, as well as becoming a shade-creating competitor of the grass needed to feed the livestock that would soon become New Zealand's economic means of survival.

As New Zealand agriculture developed a more scientific approach, field trials were conducted on how to reduce manuka, either through hard grazing or the use of powerful weed sprays.

Techniques were developed to roll over and crush manuka most efficiently with those big Caterpillar tractors, and reports were issued by a government Official Committee on Manuka Control. Manuka was called 'the arch-criminal weed' of pastures, and was said to have a significant negative impact on the national economy. One commentator insisted that 'every plant must be destroyed together with its seed' if hill-country farming was to succeed.*

Manuka even became the subject of one of the earliest examples in New Zealand of biological control. In 1937 in the mid-Canterbury region, manuka plants were discovered that appeared to be dying from some sort of disease. The leaves and trunks looked almost as though they had been blackened by fire. Within a decade observers stated that it was difficult to find any live manuka in South Canterbury. A study of the plants found several species of the sap-feeding scale insect called *Eriococcus*, an Australian native insect that presumably had been accidentally introduced, but without the natural enemies that seemed to keep it in check in its original home. And just like New Zealand honeydew on mountain beech trees, the black coloration was caused by a sooty mould fungus that lived on sap excreted by the scale insect. What was unclear was whether the sooty mould killed the manuka as a result of covering its leaves, or whether the scale insect deprived the plant of nutrients. All that was certain was that the plant died from this *manuka blight*, often within a couple of years.

As you can imagine, word spread amongst farmers in other parts of New Zealand. Infected manuka was offered for sale, and it was taken to the North Island where the disease quickly established. By 1954 it was well-distributed throughout both islands, and thousands of acres of the plant had succumbed.

But it is hard to keep a highly adaptable, genetically variable species down for long, and by the 1960s manuka had begun to recover, helped by the emergence of a pest of the pest, a fungus that attacked the scale insect. Today sooty mould can still be found on manuka, both in the wild and when it is grown as a garden ornamental, and scale insects can still be found. But the widespread presence of the death-producing species called *Eriococcus orariensis* appears to be a thing of the past.*

Manuka bee

It almost goes without saying that when you destroy something as widespread as manuka, either by blight or Caterpillar tractor, you don't just kill a plant. You also eliminate both food and shelter for a range of other species. At the level of the very small there are root fungi found in association with manuka that help with the establishment of seedlings of native beech. These *mycorrhizas* are partners that help the plants take up phosphorus, an important nutrient. Larger species found in association with manuka include a rare orchid called *Gastrodia minor* that also likes those same mycorrhizas, and a dwarf, leafless mistletoe (*Korthalsella salicornioides*). Manuka also attracts a range of insects in addition to honey bees. The plant certainly has its pests, apart from scale insects, including manuka beetles, a leaf-feeding moth, and wood borers.

However, it is in providing food from its flowers that manuka really excels. It produces both bisexual and male flowers on the same plant, and flowering is brought on by temperature and day length. There is generally a flush of flowering, but plants are also known to flower sporadically afterwards, and wild plants in some locations even seem to flower out of sequence with others elsewhere in the general vicinity.

When in full flower, you will find all sorts of flying insects on manuka, but there does seem to be a sequence, beginning in the early morning and carrying on to night. Large flies come in at dawn, followed by bees once the flowers warm up. In the evening, moths and those very long-legged insects called crane flies take up roost. In the early spring, if manuka is flowering and other plants are not, you are even likely to see monarch butterflies feeding on the nectar and sunning themselves on the top branches.

New Zealand of course has three genera, or groupings, of native bees, and at least one of those groupings, called *Leioproctus*, has a close relationship with manuka (although it likes other native and introduced flowering plants as well). There are thought to be 18 species of *Leioproctus*, and like all solitary bees, they don't live in a colony, share work, or have queens and workers. But while they might not be social insects, scientists refer to them as *gregarious*, since they make their nests in close proximity to one another.* New Zealanders may not know the bees' scientific name, and in fact

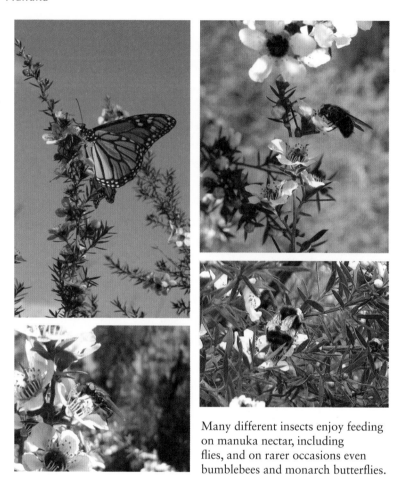

Many different insects enjoy feeding on manuka nectar, including flies, and on rarer occasions even bumblebees and monarch butterflies.

there doesn't seem to be any common one, but that hardly matters. Everyone in the country has seen them, and can usually remember as inquisitive children watching the bees fly in and out of small holes in clay banks or hard-packed sand. They are small, shiny black, and flit around much faster than bees or even wasps. Like similar ground-nesting bees elsewhere in the world, *Leioproctus* dig these holes (actually branched tunnels sometimes a third of a metre long) as a protective place in which to lay their eggs. Once the excavation has been completed, the bee heads for the flowers and collects large loads of pollen on its back legs, just the way honey bees do.

Leioproctus bees don't spend much time supping nectar, though, since they only need small amounts to fuel their activities, and to help stick together the individual pollen grains into bigger pellets.

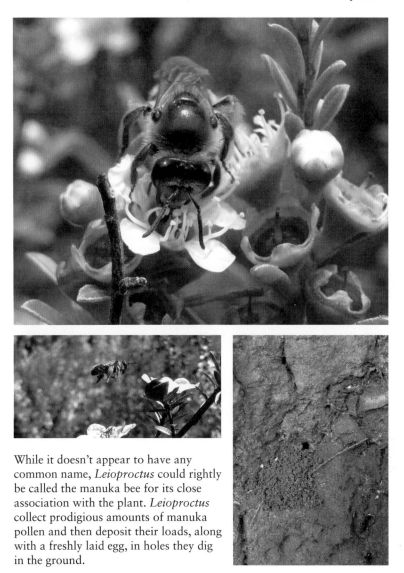

While it doesn't appear to have any common name, *Leioproctus* could rightly be called the manuka bee for its close association with the plant. *Leioproctus* collect prodigious amounts of manuka pollen and then deposit their loads, along with a freshly laid egg, in holes they dig in the ground.

The important thing is to gather lots of those flower-produced packages of protein, vitamins and minerals needed as food for their larvae. When it has a full load, the female bee flies back to its individual tunnel entrance (and we can only presume it leaves some sort of chemical pheromone at the entrance so it can tell its own nest from its close neighbours'). If you're patient you can sometimes see a *Leioproctus* bee land and climb into its hole. What you can't watch, however, is what goes on inside. The bee unpacks its loads,

125

and, when it determines it has enough pollen stored (which in good weather takes about a day), it lays an egg, then seals it off in the tunnel with a little bit of soil. What the bee has created is a 'cell', but quite different from what you would find in a honey bee colony. There isn't any wax; just a thin, transparent material surrounding it all. There is also no royal jelly production, or direct feeding of larvae. When all the provisioning is done, the bee digs another little cell cavity in a different branch of the tunnel, and starts the whole process again. *Leioproctus* aren't nurses; they're miners.

Inside the cell, the egg hatches in about three days, and the larva spends the next 10 days feeding on the pollen, all on its own. Then, as with all bees (and many other insects), the process of change into the adult (the *metamorphosis*) begins. But in the case of solitary bees like *Leioproctus*, the prepupa (the larva just before it changes form) goes into something akin to suspended animation, and doesn't turn into a fully-fledged adult until the next spring. Once an adult, if it is a male, it looks after itself and tries to find females with which to mate. If it is a female, it digs tunnels, forages for pollen, and lays eggs.

Leioproctus are great pollinators of manuka. They make their nests nearby and often emerge from their tunnels as new adults in spring at just about the time the plants begin flowering. But for solitary bees, the name of the game is working as hard as possible to increase the population of the species for the following year. There is no need for a big energy reserve back home, or for a whole host of other bees collecting food for the big family. Honey just isn't part of the picture.

Be that as it may, *Leioproctus* and honey bees together appear to have a type of *resource partitioning*, a relationship where they both use the same manuka flowers, but for more or less different purposes. *Leioproctus* have co-evolved to greatly utilise manuka pollen, so much so that it is obvious that they can use it to fully satisfy the nutritional needs of their larvae. Honey bees, on the other hand, have developed as a species together with a big range of temperate plants. They may be honey and pollen bi-vores, but when it comes to their pollen requirements, they are most definitely omnivores. To properly satisfy their nutritional requirements, especially in relation to a full complement of amino acids, they need to collect that protein material from a range of flowering species. Observation suggests, however, that manuka is generally not one of them. You very rarely see any honey bees bringing back pellet-loads of manuka pollen to their hives.*

The variability explained

While the common definition of a weed is a plant growing where it is not wanted, manuka has nevertheless always managed to also be quite useful to New Zealanders. Just as the Maori did for centuries, settlers were quick to use manuka wood as a source of fuel for cooking and heating, as all Kiwis still sometimes do. Manuka chips these days are also the premium product used to smoke meat and fish, and are available for that purpose in many stores.

As well, those early Europeans used the straight manuka poles for spokes and rails, while simple fences were made from the brush. The wood is hard, but can't stand prolonged ground contact without rotting. Still, well-cared-for garden tools with manuka handles have been known to last at least 70 years.* Bundles of the manuka twigs and branches (known as *ti-tree fascines*) also came in quite handy when trying to firm up wet and boggy sites. Manuka was said to be preferred, since it didn't seem to decompose when placed under water. Clay was often put over the bunches to create a manageable surface. Early dairy farmers found that they could use the bales around their sheds to keep the cows from 'disappearing into the mud', while in the early 1970s in the Waikato region, excavation of the main street of Morrinsville revealed that it had originally been constructed over a road bed of ti-tree fascines.*

More recently, picking up on the medicinal properties of the plant first discovered by Maori, essential oils have been distilled from the leaves of manuka. Manuka oil (not to be confused with the tea tree oil produced in Australia from *Melaleuca*) contains over 100 different compounds, but the most important are triketones, monoterpenes and sesquiterpenes.* Research has shown that the oil is antibacterial, and can also affect the *Herpes simplex* virus. It is an antioxidant, has antifungal properties, and even acts as an insecticide. Amazingly, this last property corresponds with a discovery made in recent years that a species of New Zealand parrot uses the chewed leaves of manuka to preen itself in an effort to get rid of parasites.*

Distilling products from manuka goes back to World War II, when a small industry was developed on Kawau Island, in the Hauraki Gulf near Auckland. Because most industrial chemicals were in short supply, a plant was constructed to extract both methanol and acetone from manuka, probably the earliest example of bio-fuels production in New Zealand.*

But of course the major resource obtained from manuka was, and still is, its honey. However, as the honey's special non-peroxide antibacterial properties became well known around the world, an important question needed to be answered. As Peter Molan found quite early on in his work, not all manuka honey had high levels of that activity (and in fact it was quite lucky that the one sample Kerry Simpson used in his initial test just happened to be manuka of the right sort).

Once beekeepers started getting their manuka honey tested, they developed theories about what was causing the variability in the activity. Some thought it was the weather, while others reckoned it was the soil or nutrients. It was left to a botany student at the University of Waikato by the name of Jonathan Stephens to sort it all out, and his results were published to some fanfare in 2006. Jonathan became interested in manuka honey when as a master's student he worked in Peter Molan's lab part-time, doing the gel-diffusion assay tests used to determine the non-peroxide activity rating for samples sent in by beekeepers. He and Peter often discussed why the honey had such different levels of activity, and that eventually led him to the topic for his PhD.* Jonathan's thesis is that rarest of things these days — a scientific dissertation that is well-written and quite understandable, even to non-specialists. It also details a real detective story, showing how he systematically went about eliminating the various possibilities until he finally came up with the true cause. To top it all off, it also contains a number of coloured drawings of manuka, following on in the tradition of botanical artists such as Sydney Parkinson, who produced the first such depictions of manuka after the brief collecting trip that Banks and Solander took that first day along the shores of Poverty Bay.

Jonathan analysed numerous honey and nectar samples, and was able to exclude several alternative hypotheses regarding the source of the activity, such as kanuka (unlike manuka, it didn't grow in the swamp areas that produced high-activity honey), honeydew from the blight-causing manuka scale insect (the insect's distribution didn't correlate with the activity), and environmental factors (although average annual temperature did play a role).

On the other hand, what couldn't be denied was the fact that there were a number of distinctly different varieties of wild manuka, in northern and southern branches, and the areas where these were located were linked to the level of activity in the manuka honey that was produced. In Northland — including the vicinity where Mary Bumby set up her honey bee colonies and undoubtedly produced the first-ever manuka honey in the world — a variety called *incanum* showed high activity. And connecting further dots in our story, it is probably the same variety that is found on Great Barrier Island. Interestingly, an unnamed variety with similar characteristics and activity is also present on the west coast of the South Island. As Kerry Simpson related in the first chapter of this book, that single sample of manuka honey he used in his little project came from hives located near a swamp in the Waikato. And sure enough, the variety called *linifolium* found there also proved to be highly active. Finally, there is an unnamed variety that grows on the East Cape, the type that Banks and Solander may have collected at Poverty Bay. Researchers have found that it contains an essential oil compound called *leptospermone* that has antibacterial effects. As you might guess, Jonathan found that it also produced honey with good activity.

Plantations, carbon credits and a new lease on life

It is often said that what comes around goes around, and manuka is a case in point. It is now being given a new lease on life. In fact, 'lease' is the operative word, because, as we will see, leasing turns out to be part of a remarkable new initiative involving the plant.

While manuka is still listed as a weed on the website of Massey University, one of two major schools of agriculture in the country, even that institution now concedes the irony in what has been a decades-long struggle to control it as a troublesome pest. This is not to say, however, that there isn't already plenty of manuka in the New Zealand environment. An assessment of land cover in 2002 using satellite imagery showed that there were 1,186,200 hectares of manuka and/or kanuka in New Zealand, approximately 10% of total native vegetation cover. That figure was in fact equivalent to 9% of the country's total agricultural land.* These figures provide some perspective when assessing claims sometimes made abroad that New Zealand beekeepers couldn't possibly produce so much manuka honey, or that it couldn't be such a large percentage of the nation's total crop. There is no doubt that some honey from other floral sources ends up being sold as manuka, particularly since the price differential has become almost beyond enticing, both to beekeepers, and even more so to unscrupulous on-sellers without any connection to the industry.

Despite that, however, the fact of the matter is that on the strength of manuka honey production, New Zealand beekeepers have increased their hives by 50% in the past decade, moving many of them away from more traditional honey-production areas (and especially clover-based pasture) into apiaries in manuka/kanuka scrubland that would never have been utilised before. Indeed, in some areas of the country (such as the East Cape) the number of beehives during the manuka honey flow verges on the sort of stocking rates of eight hives per hectare normally associated with the commercial pollination of kiwifruit. The big problem these days is access, since much of that manuka/kanuka scrubland is on steep and difficult terrain. In the 150 years of agricultural development in New Zealand, manuka had to bide its time by retreating back into areas that farmers didn't think was much good for anything else. It can be so hard for beekeepers to get into some locations, in fact, that helicopters are now being employed, ferrying hives into the back country, as well as lifting out again the heavy boxes filled with manuka honey in the comb.

But even that is no longer enough. Weed or not, from the time it first came into contact with Maori all those centuries ago, manuka's prevalence or otherwise in the New Zealand environment has always been the result of its relationship with us humans. And we are now going to do something with manuka that we have learned to be very good at with many other plants: we are going to turn it into a crop.

With global warming leading to calls to reduce emissions by planting native tree and shrub species that can sequester carbon in the soil, manuka appears to be a perfect candidate. As those farmers on the East Cape found to their dismay when they long ago destroyed so much manuka on their steep hillsides, the plant provides very good erosion control. Leaves can diffuse as much as 40–50% of rainfall, soil is well bound by its roots, and, best of all, its ability to take in and hold carbon is as fast and full as plantation forests of pines.*

Erosion control programmes, carbon-trading regimes, and production of the most valuable honey in the world means that the future of manuka in New Zealand looks very bright indeed. Companies like Comvita and Manukamed have announced plans to lease land and undertake manuka plantations, and they have entered into landowner agreements with the aim of gaining income from carbon credits on poor farmland planted back into the very same type of manuka bush that grew there once before.

As well, a significant programme is under way with the help of the government to develop 'high-performance' manuka selected for its ability to produce enhanced levels of non-peroxide activity in the honey that bees collect, a scheme some have dubbed 'designer scrub'. The goal of the project is to help the manuka honey industry grow tenfold to as much as $1 billion per year. That sounds almost unbelievable, but not when you consider that with the right varietal selection and increased stocking rates of beehives, the figure can be met by converting only about 50,000 of the 1 million hectares of marginal, erosion-prone land available throughout the country.* That is just one quarter of the area the government announced it was going to put into *Pinus radiata* plantations on the East Cape back in 1992, and less than the number of hectares of old-growth manuka and kanuka it said were destined to get the chop. And yes, some of those new manuka plantations are likely to be planted back on the East Cape.

The sort of production figures for highest non-peroxide activity manuka honey touted for the future will certainly be what is required, and the honey will come from arguably the first large-scale permanent stands of a nectar source planted anywhere in the world specifically for the purposes of honey production. The reason, as we will see in the next chapter, is that there is such a strong demand for at least one use of that type of manuka honey, requiring both security of supply and stability of price, that in the future the traditional way beekeepers 'chase' a honey crop may no longer always apply.

Six

SAVED BY A
POT OF HONEY

Aaron Phipps was a delightful young man, one of those people who just naturally comes across well in front of the camera. He was full of life, and maybe even a bit mischievous, and you could see that the BBC television presenter warmed to him. But then he told his story, a tale of literally coming back from death's door, and there could be no doubt. Everyone watching that night in Britain was left completely amazed.

In the first week of January 1999, Aaron contracted meningitis C, and with it meningococcal septicaemia, in effect a poisoning of the blood brought on by the disease-causing bacterium *Neisseria meningitidis*. Blood seeped into his tissues at the extremities, and the tissue itself began to die. The pain was so severe that he was put into a controlled coma for two weeks. Finally, medical staff were forced to do the unthinkable. They amputated the ends of both of his legs and the tips of most of his fingers. But his problems were far from over. As Aaron said, 'I was left with lots of big lesions on my legs from the meningitis, which even after numerous skin grafts wouldn't heal. And my pain threshold went right down so everything, basically just touching me, was really sensitive. So even after having my dressings removed I was still having to go to theatre to get new skin grafts and things.'

The presenter, who while listening to Aaron had grimaced at the thought of it all, then asked him the obvious question: 'Did you ever get to the point where you thought, this is never going to heal?'

Aaron looked down, and you could tell he was mentally recounting the feelings he had at the time. 'Yeah, there was a point

… You just started to think, after all those months … it gets to you. You think, well, this is it, is it ever going to heal?'

There was silence on the set, but only for a second. Because Aaron quickly looked up again, cocked his head, and gave the presenter a little wink. 'And then honey came along,' he smiled.

The presenter's demeanour totally changed. 'Your reaction must have been extraordinary,' she exclaimed, 'when they told you that they were going to put honey on your wounds.'

Aaron grinned again. 'Well, it was a bit of a joke at first, because we'd tried just about everything else. Any sort of dressing you can name, we'd tried it. And then a woman called Cheryl Dunford turned up and mentioned honey. And we slapped it on there, and it done the job.'

It was the last question that provided the real stunner, though. 'How quickly did the honey work?' the presenter asked.

Aaron looked directly across to her and replied solemnly, 'After nine months with no healing, within nine weeks it was completely healed. Just like that, pretty instant. And the smell was gone as well. People don't understand that wounds have a lot of funny smells, and you start to feel a bit self-conscious. But the honey stopped it completely.' He smiled again, and said, 'I smelled sweet.'

Aaron finished the interview the way he began, positive and with a twinkle in his eye. The presenter congratulated him for having coped so amazingly well with the ordeal. His cheeky reply: 'I don't care about it, to be honest. I just laugh. I've got my new legs, they're much more springy than my old ones [the ones he had lost]. They've got a bit of a bounce in the foot. So that's it now. No single girl within a hundred miles is safe.'

No doubt everyone who was watching at home joined with the presenter, who laughed with a mixture of both joy and relief.*

These days Aaron Phipps is well known in Britain, but for a completely different reason. He is a wheelchair rugby player for the national team, and in 2012 competed in the sport at the Summer Paralympics in London. He also takes part in marathons

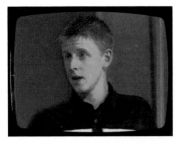

The brave and cheeky Aaron Phipps during the interview that first ignited the interest of the British public in manuka honey.

(he was ranked fourth in the London Marathon in 2009), helping raise money for a meningitis charity. He even has his own website, and an entry on Wikipedia. Back in 2000, though, as health products retailers in the United Kingdom quickly discovered, he was that young chap on telly who was literally saved by a pot of honey. But not just any honey — a remarkable one from New Zealand called manuka.

Aaron's BBC interview came at the very end of a programme segment highlighting work being carried out in five hospitals in the United Kingdom using manuka honey on stubborn wounds. Included in the segment were interview clips of two patients being treated at the Wound Healing Research Unit at Cardiff University. This is where Rose Cooper, the microbiologist we met in Chapter 4, had been testing manuka honey for its activity against the species of bacteria normally found in wounds.

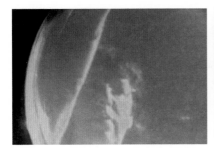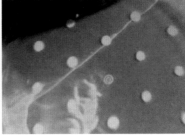

Rose Cooper showing the difference in growth of antibiotic-resistant bacteria when manuka honey has been added to the culture (no growth) and when it has not.

One of the patients was a woman with a leg ulcer that hadn't responded to normal treatments like steroids and antibiotics. She had just begun using the manuka honey, and she reported that the wound was a lot cleaner, was no longer infected, and the pain had been reduced.

Another had had a skin graft and four operations to cure a wound under her arm. But for years it wouldn't heal. Then the clinic applied manuka honey, and within three days she said 'there was a dramatic difference to the pain and what I could do, and within three months the wound was actually healed. After three years of hell, within three days my life just turned around.' She concluded by saying that it was going to be the first time in four years that she would be able to go on holiday with her young children and go swimming.

Rose Cooper was also interviewed about her research into antibiotic 'super bugs'. She said that manuka honey with good levels of non-peroxide activity killed these types of bacteria even at low concentrations, and she saw 'two patients colonised with MRSA [methicillin-resistant *S. aureus*], who once they were treated with the honey the super-bugs disappeared.' The camera showed Rose peering through some gel-diffusion plates that microbiologists use to grow bacteria. The voice-over told viewers that, with a solution of just 3% manuka honey with good levels of the activity, 'The bugs are gone. It's killing the super-bugs.'

However, the story of how manuka honey ended up being used in the Cardiff wound healing unit, and finding its way into the hands of Cheryl Dunford, that dedicated woundcare nurse who treated Aaron, begins back in New Zealand. And once again it has a lot to do Peter Molan. Not only did he discover a special non-peroxide type of antibacterial activity never seen before in honey, his inquisitiveness and enthusiasm would now also play a major role in getting the medical profession to become interested in manuka honey for use in woundcare.

A remedy re-discovered

The idea to use manuka honey in woundcare first came to Peter Molan through his brother Chris, a GP in Britain. Chris was reading through his professional publications, and knowing of Peter's new-found interest in honey, sent him an editorial he had come across in the *Journal of the Royal Society of Medicine*, one of the world's leading medical journals. The article was entitled 'Honey — a remedy rediscovered', and detailed, along with honey's ancient uses as a medicine, quite recent work on its antimicrobial properties. It also made reference to several papers in medical journals detailing its 'proven value in treating infected surgical wounds, burns and *decubitus ulcers* [pressure ulcers and bed sores].' The authors concluded with the comment that, while the actual way honey worked in some medical areas certainly needed further investigation, 'the time has now come for conventional medicine to lift the blinds off this "traditional remedy" and give it its due recognition'.*

As Peter tells it, up to that point he had just been interested in why honey was antibacterial. But when he saw the paper referring to various published articles around the world saying that honey worked on wounds that weren't healing otherwise, 'I started seeing some potential usefulness for our findings.'

What Peter did next was a lot of reading. Today science researchers can use the internet to quickly search vast databases of research, and download journal articles as PDFs. But back then he had to collect relevant literature the more painstaking way, using the services of libraries that might subscribe to the science and medical journals he was interested in. And of course every article would include references to other articles, sometimes in fairly obscure publications. But as we will see in a few pages, having to travel around searching out obscure references turned out to be very important for a couple of other reasons as well.

Even at an early stage, however, Peter was able to put together a remarkable collection of both case studies and clinical trials using honey to treat a wide range of burns and wounds. All the ones on problem wounds carried the same message, according to Peter: 'Nothing else was working, and honey did. And that seemed quite exciting from a humanitarian point of view. That's part of my nature, to help people.'

It was then that the old urge that had led him to take apart his parent's clock kicked in again. He needed to find out how the body attempted to heal wounds, and just as importantly what was it in honey that made it so special as a treatment. As it turns out, a lot of it has to do with the way honey bees transform nectar into that concentrated energy food that won't spoil. When bees 'cook' their food, this process of preservation produces some special benefits that can be especially useful to humans in a very 'unfoody' way.

The amazing self-repairing body

The human body is amazing, and the more we study it the more remarkable it reveals itself. In our cells there are believed to be millions of different substances, and while scientists are learning new things about these substances every day, they have so far identified only a fraction of them, much less come to a complete understanding of what many of them do. In fact, as one of the most comprehensive textbooks on the subject makes clear, we still know more about the structure of the universe than we do about the cells inside us.*

On more of a systems level, however, we are now well aware that our bodies constantly have to cope with incursions of potentially disease-causing organisms. Only 1 in a 1000 of these species of microbes falls into that category, but together they are still the third-largest cause of death in humans. So in an attempt to fend them off, our bodies produce an intricate set of molecules, along with a wide range of purpose-built cells and cellular processes, which together we call our *immune system*. It's a real battle, though. Pathogens (particularly viruses and bacteria) are very good at changing rapidly, and so they can sometimes avoid the effects of parts of the immune system. In complex organisms such as humans, however, there are multiple mechanisms that provide layers of defence against pathogen attack. In common with plants, we have several important layers of protection, including physical barriers (such as skin in animals, or bark in plants) and chemicals (such as acids and enzymes in the saliva and stomachs of animals, and substances in the leaves and bark in plants, all of which are always present).

We also both have an *innate immune system*, a series of responses not specific to any particular pathogen, but which occur quickly and slow up the process of infection. There is a big difference between the innate immune systems of plants and those of animals, however. Plants produce defence chemicals, like the ones in resin (and the ones honey bees often collect to make propolis) that create a scab over a tree wound. These chemicals need to work against all kinds of pathogens, producing a range of effects on the intruder's cells.

In animals like us, on the other hand, the innate system is more complex. One part we are all aware of is *inflammation* — the swelling, heat and pain caused by increased blood flow to the attacked or damaged area. Inflammation is triggered by chemical signals released by damaged cells. Signal types include *prostaglandins*, which produce fever and increase the size of blood vessels, and *interferons*, which trigger a series of special cells designed to attack. A common name for these attackers is *white blood cells*, but there are many remarkable types, including *macrophages*, which travel through the body in pursuit of invading pathogens; *neutrophils*, which, among other things, can create fibre webs to trap microbes; *mast cells*, which regulate the inflammatory response (and are associated with allergic reactions); and *natural killer (NK) cells*, which attack and destroy tumour cells, as well as cell that have been infected by viruses.

Finally, we also have an *adaptive immune system*, a further layer of protection that is activated by the innate system. As the name suggests, here the body 'adapts' its response by improving its ability to recognise the pathogen. An important part of the adaptive immune response is the *lymphocytes*, special types of white blood cells produced in the bone marrow.

B cells produce *antibodies*, which are proteins that identify foreign objects such as bacteria, viruses and even pollen. The antibody recognises a unique part of the object, which is called an *antigen*. When it does so, this puts a tag on the intruder, which can be quickly attacked by other parts of the system, or even destroyed by the B cell itself. There are also two types of cell that identify the tag. *Killer T cells* destroy cells that are infected with viruses. *Helper T cells* regulate both the innate and adaptive immune responses and help determine which response the body makes to a particular pathogen.

The amazing thing about the adaptive immune system is that, after the attacker has been eliminated, some B and T cells become long-lived memory cells, and they can help mount a faster and stronger attack when the need next arises. This is what lies behind *vaccination*, which 'challenges' our immune system with minute amounts of an often deactivated intruder. Our body is then able to recognise and destroy that type of intruder with great efficiency if we come into contact with the real disease-causing form again.

In addition to trying to keep out or destroy invading microbes that might cause disease, another important job of our immune system involves our body's sometimes almost-miraculous ability to repair itself, particularly when we damage or burn that first physical barrier of defence, our skin.

The first thing that happens is that our innate immune system produces inflammation, with white blood cells coming to the damaged area and starting to consume and remove damaged cells. The adaptive immune system also kicks in, as the body wages war with any microbes, and especially bacteria, that may have found their way into the wound.

The next step is for the rebuilding process to get under way. White blood cells create chemical messengers that tell the tissue cells nearby to start multiplying. The cells that make up the tubular structures that supply blood also start making new vessels to bring the essential nutrients and oxygen to the site needed by the tissue cells to grow. The ability of these vessels to repair themselves and create new ones is of critical importance in allowing all the other tissue cells to grow.

When the wound is of any depth, a framework needs to be put in place to help hold all the new tissue growth in place. This framework is made up of cells called *fibroblasts*. The skin layer itself also needs to grow back and cover the damage, and so *epithelial cells* receive chemical messages to start making lots of copies of themselves, right across the surface of the wound. Not everything always goes to plan, however. All those repair cells need to be in a moist environment, just as they do normally when they have that skin layer to keep them that way. Often the tissues at the surface of a wound dry out, however, because they are exposed to the air. The result is a scab. While the cells below are protected, the wound heals more slowly, and a scar remains at the end, since those skin cells haven't been able to grow right across.

And then there's the problem of inflammation, something which people who suffer from allergies know all too well. Inflammation is a two-edged sword. Too much for too long can be just as much of a problem as not enough. As we have seen, it's one of the first responses to infection, and creates redness, swelling, heat and pain, all caused by increased blood flow to the tissues surrounding the infection. The cell component of inflammation involves white blood cells, which move to inflamed tissue. Some ingest the invading pathogen, while others release granules that damage the invaders. They also, however, release chemicals that develop and maintain the inflammatory response, and sometimes the result is chronic inflammation.

In the case of a wound, the enzymes those cells release to break down and get rid of the damaged tissue debris can be over-produced, and as a result can start destroying the new tissue cells as well. Not only that, they also take apart the actual chemical signals called *growth factors* that tell existing tissue to produce more of those new cells. When too much of this happens, the wound becomes chronic. These *ulcers* are often the ones that just don't seem to be able to heal.

How honey heals

Historically, we have been slapping honey on our cuts and burns from well before we ever began to write things down. And as we saw in a previous chapter, when we did start to keep records it was fairly apparent to observers in many cultures that honey was able to heal.

The reasons why are quite numerous, as it turns out. When you put honey on a wound, the first thing it does is create a new barrier over all that damage. Just like skin, it keeps out potential invading microbes, and importantly it is moist as well. Bandages can also offer protection, but they generally aren't very moist, apart from the serum that the body is producing, which often leaks out of the wound. Honey, on the other hand, is more than simply moist. That serum, of course, contains many of the materials the body is producing to repair the wound, and honey also has a special feature that can help pull out that fluid from tissues below the wound itself. The area of damage generally doesn't have the ability to do it the normal way because the vessel structures are destroyed. Honey, on the other hand, being that super-saturated solution of sugar we discussed earlier, along with the osmotic pressure it creates, can draw out the serum into the site of the wound. Sometimes special pumps are actually used by medical staff to perform a similar function, but honey has that ability built in.

The other problem with dry bandages is that the new tissues the body makes to repair the wound often get caught up in gauze. Changing those dressings can sometimes be extremely painful, as Aaron Phipps chillingly described. The moist environment honey provides, on the other hand, keeps this damage to new tissues from occurring, and, as a result, numbers of clinical studies have shown that honey dressings create far less pain and fewer scars.

We also know that honey is very acidic, thanks to the enzyme honey bees add that creates gluconic acid. That acid, along with the osmotic pressure, keeps honey from spoiling. But it also has a helpful effect on wounds, as it has just the right level of pH to improve the rate at which wounds heal. It stimulates the red blood cells to release more oxygen, which is needed by all the new cells doing the repair work. At the same time, it keeps the inflammatory enzymes from going overboard, taking apart new cells and the substances that white blood cells produce to trigger cell growth. Those enzymes like a pH of over 7, not the 4 or 5 you find in honey.

And of course we know that bees collect honey because it is a very nutritious food, and new cells need nutrients, too. As it turns out, honey contains levels of protein building-blocks (called amino acids), vitamins and minerals that are quite similar to those found in human blood. As well, the glucose in honey is used by white blood cells to create the *respiratory burst* needed to destroy bacteria.

It has also long been known that wounds need to be cleaned, both of dead tissue, and also of the pus that is produced. If that doesn't happen, the wound often remains red and swollen, because the body's inflammation response remains in top gear. Honey is what is known as a *debrider*, a material that loosens up the dead tissue so that it can be removed, and absorbs the pus (using that sponge-like osmotic pressure again).

And then there is the other feature of honey and wounds that Aaron Phipps spoke about: its ability to eliminate the sometimes very off-putting odours that festering tissue can emit. This isn't something that is often discussed in polite company, but it is a real issue for both patients and medical staff, and honey has been found to be superior to other pharmaceutical compounds in deodorising wounds. The reason, it turns out, is the glucose in honey, which the odour-producing anaerobic bacteria prefer to the proteins they break down in the wound. When they have the option, the bacteria prefer to feed on the glucose, and the by-products then resulting from those bacteria don't give off a bad smell.

Finally there is the antibacterial effect of honey itself. The serum the body produces to feed tissue growth is also, unfortunately, a rich nutrient broth for the growth of bacteria. As we have seen, the enzymes and processes bees use to make honey keep virtually anything from being able to live in it. Bacteria don't like the acidity, which keeps them from growing. The osmotic pressure of honey is also so strong that it literally sucks the insides out of bacteria and fungi, and even out of their spores unless they have a very strong shell. Finally, when honey becomes diluted to the point where spores of sugar-tolerant yeasts can grow, the glucose oxidase, which the bees added during the curing process, kicks in, producing hydrogen peroxide, a very antibiotic substance.

It is almost as though the honey itself was part of the barrier and chemical side of the immune system. There are some problems with regular honey, though. The honey can act as a barrier, keeping out bacteria. However, while the acidity can be a help in deterring bacteria that might have already got in, once the honey is diluted by the serum being produced in the wound, it loses this antibacterial effect. Similarly, while the osmotic pressure of this super-saturated sugar substance can certainly deal to bacteria, when the honey is put on a wound it becomes diluted. Nonetheless, many bacteria cannot handle the pressure, even when honey becomes diluted to 1 to 10 with liquids like serum. However, the dreaded *Staphylococcus aureus*, the most common bacteria infecting wounds, can manage to stay alive at concentrations of honey three times that amount.

The release of hydrogen peroxide is also a much better way of dealing to bacteria than putting the chemical directly on the wound itself, as hydrogen peroxide in a concentrated form can burn new tissue. In the case of honey applied to wounds, on the other hand, the serum starts to dilute the honey, and when it reaches about 50% the moisture sets off the glucose oxidase. The action of the enzyme increases dramatically (2500 to 50,000 times), producing a constant but non-burning flow of hydrogen peroxide at a lower level (about 240 times less than in the 3% hydrogen peroxide found in standard antiseptic).

There are, however, several issues with what is this major antibacterial effect in all honeys. First, once diluted, honey only produces the substance for 24 to 48 hours, with the hydrogen peroxide ending up having a negative effect on the glucose oxidase itself. What that means, in effect, is that for normal honey dressings to have a good effect against bacteria, they need to be changed on a daily basis.

Secondly, the serum fluid that the body is making to help grow new tissue starts to dilute it, while introducing catalase, the same substance Peter Molan and Kerry Simpson added to honey back when they did the original experiment that found non-peroxide antibacterial activity in manuka honey. Catalase is actually made by our body, and is in both our cells and our serum. It deactivates hydrogen peroxide, just as it did in that experiment.

Thirdly, not all honey is the same when it comes to glucose oxidase, and therefore hydrogen peroxide production. Numerous laboratory studies have found that there can be a hundred fold

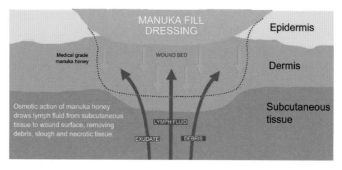

The osmotic pressure of honey draws out serum from below the wound, and acts as a debrider, loosening up dead tissue. Honey also provides a moist, sterile environment. As well, honey is antibacterial, both because it's acidic and because it produces hydrogen peroxide when diluted by the body's serum. And of course manuka honey has a special activity that can kill antibiotic-resistant bacteria commonly found in wounds.

difference in peroxide-caused antibacterial activity, depending on the honey source and, more importantly, on how the honey has been processed once it has been taken from the hive.

The glucose oxidase enzyme the bees add is very sensitive to both heat and light, and when excessive and prolonged heating is applied during honey packing to give liquid honey its long shelf-life, the result can be a significant reduction in the enzyme. As well, if the honey has been packed in a clear glass or plastic container, the same destructive effect can occur. This is why all honey used in woundcare should be in the controlled granulation form that doesn't require significant heating, and why the containers it comes in should either be non-transparent tubes or heavily-tinted jars.*

It also goes almost without saying that manuka honey with high levels of non-peroxide antibacterial activity (case and clinical studies normally use 12+) can be more effective than honey that only produces hydrogen peroxide, since manuka's special activity is heat-stable, and is not adversely affected by catalase.*

Resistant bacteria and the one-two punch

Honey is a great wound dressing, but it went out of favour with the advent of modern antibiotics. The 'wonder drugs' were seen as the solution to bacterial infections in wounds and burns, even though gauze bandages and antiseptic ointments didn't necessarily produce either the fastest or the best results. Honey, on the other hand, was capable of doing two things together that modern systems of woundcare could not — provide a moist environment required for the best tissue re-growth, while at the same time ensuring that the environment remained sterile, and in fact killed any bacteria that might venture in.

In modern medicine, you could do one or the other. You could create that moist environment, but it would become infected with bacteria. Or you could use antibiotics to kill that bacteria (sometimes very high-powered antibiotics, and at a strong dose, because the bacteria you were trying to destroy are very good at developing resistance to those drugs). But in doing so, the drugs themselves could become part of the problem. They could be so destructive to cells that they literally burned the skin, holding back the work of tissue regrowth that the body is generally programmed to do. Eventually the body might start to take no for an answer, and wouldn't properly heal itself.

The change to our view about honey as a therapeutic substance came about, however, when bacteria resistant to those wonder drugs began appearing in wounds, and the wounds refused to heal. It seemed obvious that manuka honey with high levels of non-peroxide antibacterial activity could deliver the one-two punch: kill the bacteria, and provide a great environment for tissue re-growth.

Peter Molan tried to get medical people interested in using manuka honey in woundcare, particularly when other treatments weren't working. His searches of the medical journals made it quite clear that honeys even without manuka's special properties were healing those sorts of wound. As Peter remembers, 'I tried telling people in the medical profession about what I'd found in the literature and they just said, "Oh, they would have gotten better of their own accord." That was the general reaction; I couldn't get anyone to take it seriously. At the same time I started reading more about wound healing, the biology of it, the clinical aspects of it, and realised how much people were suffering. I could see it was unnecessary suffering.'

So Peter and his graduate student Dawn Willix looked at the effect of honey on the seven most common species of bacteria found in wounds, testing for both peroxide and non-peroxide activity, and at a range of dilutions. All species were completely inhibited at 11% concentration, while manuka honey with non-peroxide activity was effective against *Staphylococcus aureus*, the most common wound species, at just 1.8% honey concentration.*

Peter also looked at strains of the super-bug methicillin-resistant *S. aureus* (MRSA), and found that non-peroxide activity manuka completely stopped its growth at 10% honey concentration. Later he and Kerry Allen, his dedicated lab assistant, found that the same applied to vancomycin-resistant *Enterococci* (VRE).*

Finally, Peter collaborated with Rose Cooper at the Wound Healing Research Unit in Wales. She looked at 58 strains of *S. aureus* isolated from infected wounds. Minimum concentrations at which all bacteria strains were inhibited was 2–3% for manuka honey and 3–4% for pasture honey. The effect was caused by factors in addition to the sugar in the honey, since the honey prevented the growth of *S. aureus* at a rate seven- to fourteen-fold greater than the concentration point where the moisture-absorbing ability of sugar ceased.

Cooper and Molan also looked at *Pseudomonas* bacteria isolated from infected wounds. *Pseudomonas aeruginosa* is an important pathogen of chronic wounds and burns, and is present in a third of all chronic leg ulcers. The bacteria are also often found in extensive burns, and reduce healing in skin grafts. The minimum inhibiting concentration for all the strains was 5.5–8.7% for manuka honey with an average non-peroxide activity. The study concluded that this type of manuka honey would prevent the growth of pseudomonas on the surface of a wound even if the honey was diluted more than tenfold by serum seepage from the wound.*

According to Peter, 'Once we began showing that the manuka honey was effective against the problem organisms, those common infective species in infected wounds, then we started getting some clinical interest.'

The first modern honey-based medicine in the world

Sabbaticals are an important and often welcome part of any scientist or teacher's career. The public sometimes thinks they are some sort of luxury, especially if the person is a university lecturer and taxpayer money is involved. But sabbaticals aren't designed to let people 'kick back'. And in the case of the ever-energetic Peter Molan, the study leave he took in 1997–1998 proved to be instrumental in manuka honey beginning to be taken seriously in the modern field of woundcare.

At the beginning of that period, he went off to two places that held extensive archives of research on honey. The first was the International Bee Research Association in Cardiff, the city of his birth. Founded by the grand dame of honey bee science, Eva Crane, for years it had the best collection of beekeeping papers and journals anywhere in the world. While he was in Cardiff, he also made sure to meet up with Rose Cooper, and together they had further discussions on the work they were both doing testing manuka honey on wound-infecting bacteria. As we will see, that meeting was very fortuitous indeed, most especially for Aaron Phipps.

Peter also went to Brisbane to meet with Dr Peter Wragg, a consultant vascular surgeon at a local hospital who was using honey as a wound dressing. He also visited Capilano Honey Ltd, the largest honey processor in Australasia. They had an excellent collection of literature on honey, including some publications Peter couldn't find anywhere else. At Capilano he met Anthony Maloney, the company's research manager. Australia produced a bit of manuka honey, from Tasmania and a few areas on the continent's east coast. They also had jelly bush, *Leptospermum polygalifolium*, and beekeepers collected some honey from that as well. Jelly bush had been tested and also showed good non-peroxide antibacterial activity.

Peter believed that manuka honey with good non-peroxide activity should be selling in pharmacies on the same shelves as antiseptics and at antiseptic prices, rather than on supermarket shelves. But he just couldn't seem to get anyone in New Zealand to take up the opportunity. For one thing, the regulatory hurdles were a big problem, as Peter and Bill Floyd found out that day in Wellington when they came up with the idea for the UMF trademark. Anthony Maloney was quite keen, however, and he had the backing of a very large honey company. Capilano formed a venture called Medihoney, and managed to succeed in getting honey registered in Australia by the Therapeutic Goods Administration. It was a tube of blended manuka and jelly bush honeys, sterilised by irradiation to ensure that not even spores of those sugar-tolerant yeasts could survive, and it was the first modern honey-based woundcare product in the world. On a gram-for-gram basis, Medihoney sold for 200 times the price of manuka honey in the jar.*

In March 1998, Peter was back in Brisbane to give a talk on manuka honey and its potential use as a dressing on wounds infected with MRSA, at the 2nd Australian Wound Management Association Conference. It would be one of over 70 such presentations he would make during his career. In this case he took a week's annual leave, going over at his own expense.

Peter vividly remembers what happened. 'I had tried writing to Waikato Hospital [his local hospital in Hamilton] and asking if they would be interested in doing a trial, but just got a polite fob-off. So I went to the conference in Brisbane, and at the end of my talk I said, "If anyone here is interested in giving manuka honey a try clinically, please catch up with me at the end of the paper. I'd love to hear from you." One person came up at the end, and said she was keen to give it a go. I asked her, where are you from? And she said Waikato Hospital. That person was Julie Betts.'

Angels that treat our wounds

It has always been said that nurses are angels of mercy. The doctors sit at the top rung of the medical ladder, but it is the nurses who do the really hard and relentless work, caring directly for the sick and injured, changing their dressings, and trying to relieve their pain.

That is certainly the case with woundcare. If you have ever looked at pictures of a gaping wound or fetid bedsore, you know that dealing with it takes a strong stomach. So try to imagine for a moment what is involved in treating those wounds, as well as investigating how the body goes about trying to heal them, especially when all efforts just don't seem to work. There are very few people in the community with that combination of both skill and dedication. In other words, as Peter Molan says, there are very few people like Julie Betts.

Julie started out as a community nurse, going into the homes of patients who required ongoing care, and, as she says, in that role, 'I got interested in woundcare because we had people with non-healing wounds and there was very little to offer them at that point in time. It wasn't that it was ignored, it was just that health professionals under-estimated it. If you had a chronic wound, you sometimes had to be home every day for a district nurse to come and dress it. So the wounds were having a huge impact on people's lives.'

These days, Julie is a nurse practitioner specialising in woundcare in one of the biggest hospital districts in New Zealand. What that means is that her skills and training are so well recognised within the health system that she has been endorsed by the Nursing Council, and is therefore able to prescribe medicines, order diagnostic tests, and set up clinics and direct treatments independently of doctors. She works with district and community nurses who provide ongoing services to patients, since very little continuing wound treatment is done in hospitals. The demand for bed space is high, so patients are sent home and cared for there. Julie is the person healthcare professionals come to when their patients have wounds that don't respond to standard forms of treatment. So it was little wonder that Julie approached Peter Molan at the conference. A product that was being reported to heal the sort of persistent wounds she was seeing more and more must have seemed like a godsend.

It didn't become obvious right away, however. It was part of Julie's reading and learning process as much as it was Peter's. She had heard him speak twice, the first time being several years before the Brisbane conference. 'That first time I thought he was mad,' she says, 'that he was definitely from another planet. But the second time I heard him speak, two years later, he'd done more research about the level of activity of honey that was required to kill bacteria, and that was the bit that made me think we might be on to something.'

At the time the whole discipline of woundcare was actually going through substantial change. According to Julie, 'We had very little in the way of methods to control bacteria in chronic wounds, so people would be on a seesaw of infection, antibiotics, okay for a couple of weeks, infection. They were on a roller-coaster ride. So I thought if you could actually manage that bacterial burden over the long term, you might tip the scales enough for the wound to heal. And I wanted to test that with honey.'*

The sort of wounds Julie is called upon to deal with don't just create serious pain and discomfort for patients; they often become debilitating and sometimes even life-threatening. Leg ulcers are a good example. These can develop in older people with poor circulation, and in people suffering from diabetes. Trying to get the tissue to re-grow is one thing, but the wounds regularly become non-healing because they become infected with antibiotic-resistant bacteria. And the prognosis isn't good. There is such a high risk of the bacteria getting into the bloodstream, with resulting blood poisoning of the sort Aaron Phipps suffered from, that amputation sometimes becomes the only recourse. In the United States, for instance, about 50% of all non-traumatic leg amputations are due to infected diabetic ulcers. Even with that drastic treatment, however, five-year mortality rates for those patients range between 39 and 68%.

A.k.a. Jem Bonnievale

In some of the original work Julie was involved with at Waikato Hospital, the manuka honey was administered straight onto these sorts of ulcers and then covered with gauze. Staff were pleased with the results on about a dozen such chronic wounds, but Peter wasn't. He realised that when the honey was heated by the patient's body it started to run off. Nursing staff, who are always rushed off their feet, also wanted a more user-friendly product; something they could rip out of a packet and slap on as they were used to doing with other dressings.

The wound dressing Peter came up with couldn't have been more basic. It was just standard *gamgee tissue*, a thick layer of absorbent cotton wool between two layers of absorbent gauze. The gamgee was invented in 1880, but it is still a mainstream dressing today. The dressing was put in a plastic bag, and then manuka honey with good non-peroxide activity was added. The entire process was carried out in a pharmaceutical manufacturing facility, audited under the worldwide Good Manufacturing Practice (GMP) system.

The first batch had a bit of a problem, however. The manufacturer put in 5 grams more honey than Peter had wanted. He wasn't aware of the problem, however, until Julie came to him with complaints from patients. When they put the honey-impregnated pads under a pressure bandage on their leg ulcer, the tension from the bandage was squeezing out that extra honey, and it oozed down their legs and into their shoes!

The dressings certainly worked, however. The second batch — this time with the right amount of honey — made its way over to Rose Cooper in Cardiff. And it was Rose who supplied another angel of mercy: Cheryl Dunford, the nurse Aaron Phipps talked about in that BBC interview. Cheryl performed a role similar to Julie's in the Salisbury District Hospital, in the southwest of England. She advised on the care and management of patients with what are called *complex wounds*, and part of her job was to look for and trial new products that might work with wounds that won't heal.

Cheryl was called in by nursing staff who were gravely concerned for Aaron's well-being, since, besides the problems with the six skin grafts he had received in an attempt to cover over his amputation wounds, he had also developed a bed sore. Swabs from his various lesions were cultured, and it was found that the wounds had major infections of *Pseudomonas*, *S. aureus* and *Enterococcus*.

They had tried all manner of dressings, and while multi-layered bandages seemed to help clean the wounds, the need for constant changing, and the pain they created as the gauze stuck to the tissue, became, according to Cheryl, 'traumatic for all concerned'.

Luckily she had read the papers by Rose Cooper and Peter Molan showing that the very same bacteria infecting Aaron's wounds were highly susceptible to manuka honey, so she contacted Rose for advice. What she got in return were Peter's honey-impregnated dressings. The results were dramatic, to say the least. Cheryl went on to report Aaron's case in a leading nursing journal in the United Kingdom, using the patient name 'Jem Bonnievale' to protect Aaron's privacy. Aaron, on the other hand, wasn't that concerned.

He was happy to be interviewed directly about what seemed to be almost a miracle.*

Cheryl's case study reports, along with Aaron's interview, generated enormous publicity for manuka honey in Great Britain. As Bill Bracks, who was with Comvita at the time, remembers, all their manuka honey vanished off the shelves of retailers in the United Kingdom almost overnight after Aaron's appearance on television, and the company had to air-freight pallet-loads of manuka honey in an attempt to meet the demand.

A dressing for awkward places

For those people who are important enough in this world to be interviewed, whether it be in the print media or on television, there is always the fear of being misquoted or, even worse, having the film editors pick a shot that you thought was going to

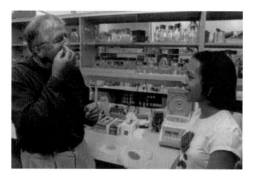

The screenshot of Peter Molan showing the BBC interviewer how his honey alginate dressing is so pliable you can stick it up your nose!

definitely be an 'out-take'. Peter Molan certainly had a small problem of that kind when a segment appeared on the BBC programme *Tomorrow's World* in 2001.

The programme once again detailed the woundcare properties of manuka honey, including an interview in New Zealand of a patient who had a sore on his foot that had turned into a wound that wouldn't heal for over three years. As he said, the honey was the only thing that made any difference. Back in the lab, Peter then showed the reporter a manuka honey wound dressing that had been put onto an agar plate inoculated with bacteria. He held it up and it was obvious from the clear ring around the dressing that the honey was keeping the growth of the bacteria at bay.

It was certainly a unique dressing. It didn't seem to be on any gauze or bandage, but at the same time it also wasn't runny. It looked for all the world like a big piece of fruit leather. Peter showed how it stayed together as he grasped it at one end and moved it up and

Saved by a pot of honey

down. Next, he told the interviewer how it could be put into awkward places, bending it so that it fit in the webbing between two of his fingers. Then the reporter asked another question about the consistency of the product. Peter explained that it could be made harder or thinner or more stretchy. As a demonstration he broke a piece off, and then while saying that you could shape it and put it in hard-to-reach places, he did something almost without thinking … he stuck it up his nose.*

The next day he received an email from his brother Chris, the GP, who had watched the programme in Britain the night before. The email read simply: 'Well, at least you didn't show her how to use it to treat piles!'

Making honey like rubber

Everyone had a laugh at the BBC segment, but the new dressing Peter Molan had now shown everyone was very serious indeed. In fact, it was something of a world first. As the *Tomorrow's World* presenter put it, making honey into a solid form suitable for a dressing had never seemed possible before.

As Peter tells it, he and the woundcare nurses led by Julie were on a 'steep learning curve. The dressings we made were sticky, and the honey was getting flushed away by the wound fluid, so we sometimes ended up with just plain cotton wool against the wound. I wanted something better than that. We needed to get the honey into a non-runny form that was easy to handle, and that would absorb fluid without the honey getting washed away.'

It turned out to be a case of 'thinking about it a lot', as well as conducting a number of experiments in his kitchen at home. Peter tried all sorts of gelling agents. Eventually he stumbled on alginate, a powdered product extracted from seaweed. Dentists use it to make teeth moulds. It didn't work in the honey at first, but eventually he sorted out the process by warming the mixture. 'I came up with a way of making the honey like rubber,' he recounts. 'You could have it from something that almost looked like honey, to a gel you could put in a tube, to something really firm.'

The invention was patented by the University of Waikato, mostly to ensure that it would be taken through the process of registering it as a medical product. As Peter says, he has never sought any personal financial gain from his discoveries about manuka honey and wound healing. But the alginate wound dressing did work its way through the business world, first with a small company in the Waikato town of Cambridge called Bee & Herbal, then on to Comvita, who eventually acquired both Bee & Herbal and the Medihoney brand from Capilano. Finally both the brand and the dressings were passed on to Derma Sciences, a mainstream woundcare company in the United States.

It was — and very much still is — a joint venture, with Derma Sciences having access to and credibility within the mainstream medical establishment, and Comvita being able to supply the manuka honey that is needed. Comvita has sophisticated quality assurance and auditing systems, as well as beehives that can produce and supply medical-grade manuka honey, using one of the most modern and hygienic honey extraction and processing plants you will see anywhere. It can standardise the product so that every batch has the same level of non-peroxide antibacterial activity.

As the market for the wound dressings develops, Comvita is investing in tens of thousands more of its own beehives, running them under highly audited GMP systems, and developing plantations of selected varieties of manuka to produce nectar that its bees will make into high-activity honey. The goal, which in fact is an absolute necessity, is to create a steady and increasing supply at a price not determined by the honey's rapidly increasing demand elsewhere in the marketplace. It is an important reason that manuka in New Zealand has that 'new lease' on life.

A helping honey in a zone of war

We are in what looks like a shed used to repair and store vehicles, with a 5-metre high slanted corrugated-iron roof and bare plywood walls. It wouldn't be out of place on most New Zealand farms. But this one is full of frantic parents and children crying out in pain. Burly young men with short haircuts and desert-camouflage fatigues move hurriedly among the throng, wearing surgical rubber gloves. It quickly becomes obvious that this is not some quiet barnyard; it is instead a massive fuel depot, the men are security personnel who normally protect armed convoys, and they are offering their services as medical volunteers while they wait for their next trip. It's a bit like *M*A*S*H*, only one step up from tents.

Welcome to the Smith Gate Burn Clinic, the only specialist paediatric burn unit in war-torn Iraq. The scenes all around are enough to bring even the most battle-hardened soldier to tears. A boy displays horrible red scars covering almost all of his back. Another child cries out in pain as a volunteer from the 82nd Airborne Division, Sergeant Joe Barzeski, removes the loose, dead skin from an 11-year-old with massive burns. He has to turn up the radio that is playing nearby to drown out the child's cries. The clinic doesn't have any pain-relieving drugs. But they still manage to treat up to 80 patients a day.

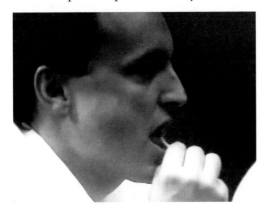

A screenshot of Dr Ted Fogarty taking a bite of Medihoney alginate wound dressing, 'the only woundcare product on the market you would ever want to eat.'

You would be forgiven for thinking that these poor children are the innocent victims of the ravages of war, the most vulnerable of the people who are often forgotten in the armed conflicts that have marked our species for thousands of years. But in fact this is not the case. They are instead just children who were being playful, or helping their parents with the daily chores, and they have been burned because open cooking fires, boiling water in uncovered pots, and fragile kerosene lanterns are the norm not just in Iraq, but in many places that don't have the infrastructure that we take for granted in more developed parts of the world.

When Craig Lambrecht, a medical doctor with the North Dakota National Guard, first came to the clinic, he was both amazed at the dedication of the volunteer soldiers, and appalled at the lack of medical supplies available to them. Because the children weren't injured by any direct act of war, the US Army's rules of engagement did not allow military provisions to be used. Craig started to contact his friends and colleagues back home in an effort to get donated medical goods. That was when a doctor at the hospital Craig had worked at previously, by the name of Ted Fogarty, responded to the call. Or at least he tried. He sent Craig an email one morning at 2 a.m. about a new type of woundcare product he had come across on the internet. But as Craig recalls, 'I'd never heard of it … so I ignored him, and I ignored him for a couple of weeks.'

That product did make its way to Smith Gate Burn Clinic, however. In fact, Ted Fogarty went on to spend several thousand dollars of his own money buying and shipping it. And when it arrived it certainly changed Craig's mind: 'Literally within the first week it changed the way we provided burn care to our children. And the old white *silvadene* [silver sulfadiazine ointment, the standard burn treatment] was pretty much on the way out.' The product Ted had recommended 'was our new standard'.

'It would basically help dissolve the dead skin, take the dead skin off,' according to Craig, explaining the process of debridement. And the young patients 'had less pain, they had less itching, there was better healing'.

In a segment on television back home in Bismarck, North Dakota, sometime later, he and Ted discussed the product. To the astonishment of the reporter, Ted cut off a strip of the dressing and, putting it into his mouth, began to chew.

It was Peter Molan's alginate and manuka honey discovery, now being manufactured and provided free of charge to the clinic by Derma Sciences — making a real difference in Iraq. Craig Lambrecht liked the product so much, in fact, that he has said, 'I would use the Medihoney on burns on my children, as the first choice, without question.'

It turned out that Ted Fogarty wasn't the only one who sampled the product that day in Bismarck. The presenter herself had tried it, and, while she reported that it didn't quite taste like the honey she was used to, there could be little argument that is was probably the only woundcare product on the market that you might want to eat.*

The gold standard of woundcare

There are close to two dozen honey-based woundcare products available today, manufactured by at least seven different companies, with the majority using manuka honey with high levels of non-peroxide antibacterial activity.* The reason that sort of honey is used, rather than other honeys, is simply that the special type of activity found in manuka has been shown not to be destroyed by the catalase the body produces, which is present in wound serum.

The products themselves include ointments, gels, impregnated non-adherent gauze, and polyacrylamide sheets, along with the alginate dressings, and work is being undertaken to improve design and delivery, particularly in relation to absorbing *exudite* (the serum produced by the wound). The gels have been shown to reduce the stinging sensation that is sometimes associated with honey dressings. The acidity in the honey can be detected by inflamed nerve endings in the wound, although, as Julie Betts says, it is still hard to predict who will and who will not be affected.

The need for these products is both large and growing. Worldwide, the market for products to treat *advanced wounds* — the roughly one half of all wounds that don't heal normally and persist, and the ones that first brought manuka honey to the attention of woundcare nurses — is over US$5 billion per year, and growing annually by 10%. It represents over a third of the total world woundcare market. The increase in advanced wounds is being driven by a number of factors, including increasing diabetes rates, longer life expectancy, and of course the development and spread of antibiotic-resistant bacteria.*

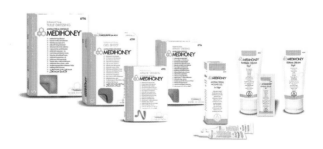

The Medihoney range, including the alginate wound dressing first developed by Dr Peter Molan.

Woundcare products including honey have become mainstream in the way that anything these days is accepted in modern medicine — government authorities have approved them for registration. As we saw earlier, that *Leptospermum* honey in a tube developed by Capilano became the first product ever registered for woundcare, when the Australian government approved it in 1999. Several years later, funding for its use was provided by the public health systems in Queensland and New South Wales. In 2004, the first commercial wound dressing using honey, produced by a British company called Advancis Medical, was granted registration by authorities in the United Kingdom, and the National Health Service began covering the cost in 2005.

Finally, in 2007 it was announced that Derma Sciences' Medihoney line of manuka honey and alginate dressings had been cleared for sales and marketing by the Federal Drug Administration (FDA) in the United States. The FDA is the most stringent regulator of medical products on the planet, and Medihoney was arguably the first bee-derived product ever to receive such clearance by that governmental authority. A number of clinical uses were listed for Medihoney, including the treatment of burns, surgical/traumatic wounds, infected surgical wounds, pressure ulcers (bed sores), venous ulcers (wounds that occur because of improper circulation in the legs), and diabetic arterial ulcers (related to nerve damage caused by diabetes).*

The FDA is considered the 'gold standard' when it comes to medical products, and many other countries around the world accept its conclusions without having to carry out any further scrutiny of the high level of data required. That sort of data includes complex clinical trials involving large numbers of patients and often significant investments by companies hoping to have their products approved, a hurdle that very few other natural products have ever overcome.

Seven

LET FOOD BE
THY MEDICINE

The New Zealand Herald is the major daily newspaper in Auckland, by far and away the largest city in the country. So when an article with the words 'health warning' in the title appears in that paper, it is fair to say a lot of New Zealanders take notice.

In November of 1997, about 18 months after Peter Molan had received his MBE for discovering the unique antibacterial activity of manuka honey, and just before he left for Cardiff on the visit where he gave Rose Cooper those wound dressings that were eventually used to treat Aaron Phipps, a press release from the New Zealand Ministry of Health was printed virtually verbatim in the *Herald*. And even the casual reader could see that it mentioned both 'health warning' and 'honey bees'. The article itself was about the ministry's decision to require mandatory label warnings regarding allergic reactions on three bee products: royal jelly, pollen and propolis. The warnings came about because of a disputed case in Australia where a coroner had blamed royal jelly for the death of a surfer who also happened to suffer from severe asthma.

Label warnings were certainly a legitimate requirement on these products, because of course everyone knows that people are allergic to pollen, whether it is collected by bees or not. And beekeepers from time to time develop dermatitis from prolonged contact with propolis. Most dietary supplements that were on sale in the country containing these products already had such warnings. More so, as it turned out, than for either peanuts or shellfish, both of which can cause severe allergic reactions that each year in New Zealand result in hospital admissions and sometimes fatalities. Despite all that, however, the truly amazing thing was a statement in the middle of the article, made under something called 'limited privilege' by the Acting Director-General of Health. This was the man ultimately responsible for the entire health system, which is the second-largest item of expenditure of public finances in the country. And his advisors had recommended that he say in print that for the bee products in question 'there was no scientifically demonstrated nutritional or medical benefit'.*

As for honey in general, and manuka honey in particular, neither were even mentioned. But as Bill Floyd and Peter Molan discovered that sunny day in Wellington when they came up with the idea that eventually became the UMF trademark, no medicinal claims could be made for those products either. Honey was in the Food Act, and you couldn't make health claims about food.

The dichotomy of Hippocrates

For anyone involved in research on the therapeutic properties of bee products, even at that time the statement by the Ministry of Health was clearly ill-informed. And as we have seen, in the following decade the medical use of honey in woundcare once again became mainstream. But what led those government health advisors, well-trained in the assessments needed to allow a medical claim of use to be put on even the lowest grade of 'pharmacy-only' products, to advise their head health bureaucrat to take such a draconian line?

Believe it or not, it goes back as far as Hippocrates, the so-called 'Father of Modern Medicine', and also has a lot to do with a split that more recently happened in Western medicine; a split that wasn't nearly as drastic in the East, and in particular China, the oldest continuing civilisation on Earth.

Although Hippocrates is such an important figure in the history of medicine, there is a lot we don't know about him. As is the case with many such luminaries from ancient times, much of what has come down to us in the present day is subject to scholarly dispute. We do know that he resided on the Greek island of Kos, was born around 460 BC, and that both his father and his sons were also physicians. It is said, as well, that he lived a long and useful life, perhaps surviving beyond the age of 100. Much of the rest, however, can only be attributed to a group that supposedly followed his teachings. Nevertheless, for the health and well-being of us all, those teachings are more than enough.*

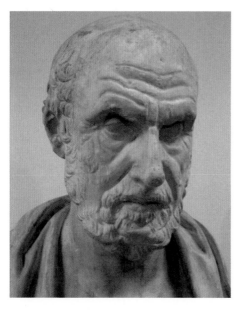

Hippocrates, the 'Father of Modern Medicine', and the author of the famous motto: 'Let food be thy medicine, and medicine be thy food.'

Before Hippocrates' time, everyone believed that disease was the result of displeasing the gods. Ever after, at least for the sensible (and as we know, the idea of what is 'sensible' has often waxed and waned), illness has been something with direct causes that can be observed, recorded, and learned from. Medicine isn't religion or philosophy; it is a practice that can be improved upon over time by carefully and humanely studying the patients themselves. Hippocrates gave the world *case records* (the objective writing down of a patient's symptoms and outcome), *prognosis* (the ability to predict the course of a disease or condition based on the careful reading of those past case records), and *diagnosis* (the attempt to identify a disease based on a knowledge of symptoms). His teachings provided the basis for what doctors still use today, namely *clinical practice*: the ability to learn from your peers and your experience, and to change your treatment of patients based on that learning, rather than falling back on ritual and superstition.

Needless to say, the medical philosophy espoused by Hippocrates didn't become ascendant immediately, and the world owes much to the Islamic civilisation for adopting his methods in the Middle Ages at a time when the Catholic Church had all but driven out the idea that sickness was caused by anything other than God's will. The rationalism and deductive reasoning inherent in the Hippocratic method really took hold in Europe during The Enlightenment, however, and the idea of clinical practice became a strong foundation for modern medicine as it developed in the nineteenth century.

These days Hippocrates is honoured in the medical fraternity in the best possible way. The oath he was said to have administered to his students has now become the basis for a pledge made by young doctors before they begin practising. Its most fundamental maxim is 'first, do no harm'. The Hippocratic Oath is a statement of ethics and the proper treatment of patients which provides a moral strength to medicine often not found in many other walks of life.

Hippocrates is also known for another saying, one that now is often seen as quite contrary to the way modern medicine is practised. The actual cures Hippocrates espoused were not the sort of interventions of drugs and surgery we take for granted today. He was said to rely on the 'healing power of nature', and as such his treatments generally involved giving the patient rest, keeping everything clean (including the doctor's hands and fingernails), and soothing the patient through the crisis that would signal whether the disease would successfully run its course.

He did, of course, use remedies that were available at the time, and as we saw in Chapter 2, he prescribed honey-based mixtures for fever, pain and wounds. But his regimes didn't involve many of the other, more potent drugs used by others, particularly since he believed that a wrong treatment given as a result of an incorrect diagnosis could in fact 'do harm'. This was the philosophy behind his famous motto: 'Let food be thy medicine, and medicine be thy food.' At the time this idea would probably have seemed obvious to everyone, and it is still a statement that makes complete sense to the Chinese. For over 2000 years that civilisation has practised medicine with what has become known as a *holistic approach*. They use an extensive array of herbal remedies, but, like Hippocrates, dietary therapy is also very important.

However, it is the other side of Hippocrates' philosophy that has provided a basis for the way modern medicine is now practised in the West. Clinical practice is still uppermost, and the sort of case reports that Hippocrates first developed now fill your GP's computer, as well as finding their way into medical journals, as we saw in the case of Aaron Phipps (a.k.a. Jem Bonnievale). Hippocrates clearly believed we could build our understanding of medicine by observation, collection of information, and analysis, so he would no doubt approve of the fact that medicine has also now become a science. We have discovered that we can learn more about best practice and what works, as well as what doesn't, by applying the scientific method, including trials on patients and test volunteers, as well as by statistical analysis to determine whether or not what was tested actually produced a valid result.

It is this sort of *evidence-based medicine* that was behind that statement made back in 1997 by the New Zealand Director-General of Health. He said there were no 'scientifically demonstrated' benefits to the products. But what he really meant, I think it is clear in hindsight, was that the therapeutic properties displayed by royal jelly, propolis and bee pollen hadn't been substantiated by the sort of clinical studies that met the standards of his advisors, a standard now being applied to all manner of compounds and practices used to treat people around the world.

Living in the dawn of evidence-based medicine

The development of manufactured antibiotics after World War II pushed the pharmaceutical industry to create more and more chemically derived (*synthetic*) compounds to be used as drugs. And at the same time, employing Hippocrates' dictum of doing no harm, regulatory authorities came up with processes that these companies needed to go through to ensure that their formulations hopefully did what they claimed they would, as well as not creating adverse effects.

But what is really interesting is just how recent all this is. The author David Bornstein has pointed out that the first randomised study of a medication (the antibiotic streptomycin) was published in 1948, and it wasn't until 1962 — after the scandal arising from the use of thalidomide, which produced birth defects in babies whose mothers had taken the drug — that the US government began requiring drug manufacturers to show 'substantial evidence of effectiveness'. The term *evidence-based medicine* itself only entered common usage in 1992.*

The process regulators use is an assessment of the quality of evidence, and they have a strict hierarchy of what sort of evidence is best. The lowest is *in vitro*, or 'test tube', studies. These show, for instance, the action of a compound against a disease-causing organism. That first gel-diffusion assay of manuka honey that Peter Molan and Kerry Simpson carried out was a basic *in vitro* study.

Next is *in vivo*, or animal studies. As we all know, guinea pigs have become so famous in testing drugs which we are not sure are effective or safe on humans, that their name has become synonymous with these sorts of animal tests.

The most basic level of human evidence is the *case report*. These shouldn't be scoffed at, although medical authorities sometimes do. As we have seen with honey and the treatment of wounds and burns, without case reports we often don't find out about new treatments, or bring back old ones, either of which might be worth investigating in a more systematic way. The famous gift to medicine that Hippocrates created in the form of the case report is just as important now as it was 2500 years ago.

However, to be allowed to make therapeutic claims, a product is generally required to show a significant effect in *clinical trials*, with *controls* (patients not receiving the drug), the use of *placebos* (patients getting something else they think is the drug, in order to eliminate psychological influences) and *double-blinds* (with neither the patents nor the persons administering the drug knowing which is the placebo and which is not). Finally, when enough clinical trials have been done there is the *meta-analysis*, where a statistical analysis of these clinical trials is carried out to determine if there is sufficient agreement among all the trials. These are then combined with the more qualitative results of things, like case reports, to provide a *systematic review*.

It is an extremely stringent process. So stringent, in fact, that it is often said that, using this sort of assessment criteria, only 20% of standard medical treatments are evidence-based. This figure is no doubt too low, since of course there are a number of procedures doctors and nurses carry out that don't need to be tested by expensive and complicated clinical trials. If someone severs an artery, you don't need a meta-analysis to know that a tourniquet will save the patient's life.

Interestingly, however, now that a number of systematic reviews have been conducted in the medical field, the results are very mixed. In 2007, an assessment was made of the work carried out by a major supplier of these reviews, the Cochrane Collaboration. (Archie Cochrane was the man who published a book in 1972 outlining the methods of evidence-based assessment.) A total of 1016 systematic reviews were analysed, and just 44% found the procedure or drug likely to be beneficial. Luckily, only 7% actually deemed the treatment to be harmful. However, virtually half concluded that the evidence didn't support either a positive or a negative effect, and almost all (96%) recommended that more research needed to be done.*

Honey as a non-alternative medicine

So what of honey, and manuka honey in particular? By far and away the greatest amount of clinical evidence exists for the use of honey in woundcare. Thanks to the interest manuka honey has generated around the world, the number of studies in this field has increased significantly since that editorial in the *Journal of the Royal Society of Medicine* in 1989, the one Peter Molan's brother sent him that called for physicians to lift their blinds and give honey the recognition it deserved.

It has taken some time, however, and some of the earlier evidence-based reviews have produced mixed results. That is not the case with the most recent systematic analysis, however, which lists 55 medical studies on burns, ulcers and other wounds, including 32 clinical trials of one variety or another. In total, over 4000 patients were involved. And 29 of those studies used manuka honey with high levels of non-peroxide antibacterial activity (including those honey and alginate dressings that Peter Molan first developed). The result of that analysis, even when applying the most stringent evidence-based criteria, was that 'honey is a dressing with properties that are beneficial to wound healing' as well as having 'antibacterial capacity'. A similar review article concluded that 'there is biologic evidence to support the use of honey in modern woundcare, and the clinical evidence to date also suggests a benefit.' As you might guess, however, based on what we have seen about how the process works, both reviews recommend that in the future more well-designed trials using larger numbers of patients should be conducted to better understand honey's therapeutic effects.*

It would seem that honey, and manuka honey in particular, is finally getting the medical acceptance it deserves. As Peter Molan says, when it comes to woundcare, honey isn't some sort of 'alternative' or 'complementary' medicine, any more than is the silvadene that the staff at the Smith Gate Burns Clinic in Iraq first used. Both were standard wound treatments before World War II, went out of favour when antibiotics came on the scene, and now have been brought back into use as a result of the development of antibiotic-resistant bacteria.* Silver dressings were the first to re-enter the market, and then had a much bigger budget for advertising and distribution. But honey — especially when it is manuka honey with high levels of non-peroxide antibacterial activity capable of killing antibiotic-resistant bacteria — has been shown in a variety of clinical studies to be comparable to, if not better than, other dressings that have now come back into vogue.

So why is it that many medical staff are still reluctant to use honey in woundcare? Part of it is simply lack of understanding of why it might work, as both Julie Betts and Dr Craig Lambrecht conceded. And as Peter Molan has pointed out, despite the 'modern mantra of evidence-based medicine', when healthcare professionals don't know how a product works there is an inclination to 'dispute the evidence rather than try the product'. Part of it may also be the tendency for natural products to often be touted as a cure-all, or magic bullet, something which physicians and nurses know from experience just isn't true. And finally, a big part of it is also a result of what modern medicine has become. We have made great progress in the past half-century in all manner of areas of healthcare, and that progress is directly aligned with everything becoming more complex and technical. It follows, then, at least for people who have been more recently trained in the field, that if it is sophisticated it must be best. A supposedly simple, or at least non-industrialised, substance like honey doesn't fit into that mould. In that sort of mind-set, it just doesn't make sense that a food can be a medicine, despite what Hippocrates might have said.

A detective novel that doesn't seem to end

Knowing how something works is what has always driven people like Peter Molan. But there are more examples than you might think of procedures and drugs being used in medicine before the precise mode of action, or even the active compound, is known. That has certainly been the case with manuka honey. Eventually, though, we need to find some answers, and that is where science-based enquiry comes to the fore.

Science-based enquiry allows us to investigate supposedly 'simple' substances like honey, and when we do we find that they are much more complicated than we thought. The worldwide popularity of manuka honey has created a renewed interest in honey in general on the part of scientists. For the medical regulators those 'test-tube' studies the scientists carry out might be at the lowest, laboratory-based rung on the evidence-based assessment ladder, but for the rest of us the resulting discoveries that are made are often nothing short of amazing.

Let's take the case of the antibacterial activity of honey. It can perhaps be likened to a detective novel, but one that becomes more and more complicated the further a particular 'line of enquiry' is pursued. And it is a process that doesn't necessarily come to an end any time soon, the way it might in a book. We certainly have the suspect, and there are more than a few dead bodies. Combining lists from several sources, and going back as far as 1919 when the very first paper on the antibacterial activity of honey was published, scientists have shown that honey is capable of inhibiting the growth of — and often killing outright — at least 100 different species of disease-causing bacteria.*

But that is not enough. What about the murder weapons? We need to know just what it is about the honey that kills the bacteria, or at least keeps it from growing. There is the acidity of the honey, but that gets diluted quite quickly, especially when it comes into contact with wounds. And there is the super-saturated sugar content, the osmotic sponge that sucks bacteria dry. It is the same reason you find so much sugar in fruit preserves; it keeps bacteria and fungi from growing and spoiling the jam. But studies have shown that even when honey is diluted over twentyfold, to the point where the osmotic effect has all but disappeared, honey still manages to knock out bacterial germs.

In fact it was an experiment involving dilution in that first paper published back in 1919 that made scientists aware that something else was involved. When honey was diluted with fetid water containing bacteria capable of causing intestinal diseases, the ability of the honey to kill the bacteria actually increased.* It took another 20 years to give the effect a name (*inhibine*), and a further two decades before the link became clear between the glucose oxidase the bees added to honey and the hydrogen peroxide it produced when the honey was diluted. And we still don't know why glucose oxidase is inactive in full-strength honey.

Then of course there was the discovery Peter Molan and Kerry Simpson made: the special property in some manuka honey that had nothing to do with hydrogen peroxide, and which made it especially useful in woundcare because it lasted longer than the 24 to 48 hours hydrogen peroxide remains in honey that has been diluted by body fluids.

But what precisely was it in manuka honey that was killing even bacteria resistant to other antibiotics, and at honey concentrations in some cases as low as 2%? You might think that these days the task of finding out would be fairly easy, particularly with the sophisticated analytical equipment scientists now have at their disposal that can identify individual chemical compounds in a substance in parts per billion. But as we will see in the next chapter, that isn't necessarily always the case. You can now take almost any substance to bits. But real skill is required, often by people in different laboratories combining their findings over time, to determine which of those bits causes the effect.

As if that wasn't hard enough, in our detective novel we also need to call in the forensic specialists (the people from *CSI*). The mystery isn't really solved until we figure out exactly *how* the weapons caused the death. How did the various physical properties and chemical compounds go about killing the bacteria, or at least stopping them from multiplying to the point where they can do real harm?

It is an intriguing investigation, since, as you may recall from that previous comment about cells versus the structure of the universe, we sometimes don't know everything about the cell processes involved. So part of our learning about those very cells can come from watching individual properties and honey compounds produce various actions, both in the work that goes on within cells and between them, as well as how those cellular actions bring about effects in bodily tissues and organs. This sort of research inevitably works its way down to the level of individual genes, which turn those processes on and off. And that is where the individual honey compounds sometimes have their ultimate impact. The detective novel can't end until we get to the very essence of life itself.

Honey, bacteria and biofilms

So far, the final chapters of how honey manages to be antibacterial read something like this: honey is directly bactericidal, but it also keeps some bacteria from doing something that helps them protect themselves. As well, honey seems to be able to keep bacteria from becoming so virulent. And interestingly, much of the most recent work in trying to understand the direct mechanisms involved has been done with manuka honey.

Killing bacteria depends on the species. In the case of the antibiotic-resistant *S. aureus* (MRSA), manuka honey stops the *cell cycle*, the way bacteria create copies of themselves. It stops the activity of *autolysins*, enzymes that digest the cell wall of the bacteria so it can burst out in the form of two cells. Manuka honey also stops a special protein in MRSA from doing its work in helping the bacterial cells cope with environmental stress. On the other hand, in *Pseudomonas* bacteria often found in non-healing wounds, manuka honey destroys the envelope of the cell itself, causing the contents of the cell to leak out and die. It actually reduces the expression of a gene that is important in maintaining the structural integrity of the cell. In *Escherichia coli* — the infamous *E. coli* that can cause food poisoning — manuka honey changed the expression of 2% (up) and 1% (down) of the bacteria's entire complement of genes.

As we know, however, bacteria are very crafty at protecting themselves, and in the past several decades researchers have started to delve deeply into one of the most important of these protection mechanisms, something called *biofilms*. Probably the best-known type of biofilm is the plaque that bacteria produce on teeth. The bacteria secrete a slime that not only protects them from enemy bacteria, but also from the immune system components contained in our salvia. As well, the slime helps bacteria stick to the surface

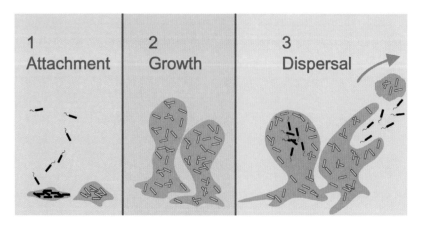

Biofilms are one of the main ways colonies of bacteria manage to protect themselves, both from competing bacteria and from human-applied antibiotics.

of the tooth, and grow together in communities that can attack the enamel and cause decay.*

Biofilms are a particular feature of disease-causing bacteria, and are thought to be involved in 80% of human infections. They also make it hard to treat these bacteria with antibiotics, probably because the drugs have a hard time getting through the slime. Studies have shown that bacteria in biofilms can be up to 1000 times more resistant to antimicrobial substances, even though the same bacteria are easily killed by those compounds when not surrounded by biofilm.* That being the case, scientists are quite excited about the discovery that manuka honey can keep biofilms from sticking, as in the case of *Streptococcus mutans*, a bacteria that causes plaque and tooth decay. And manuka honey also seems to work against multi-species biofilms in the mouth. Biofilms are also present in wounds, allowing the bacteria that produce them to persist, even when synthetic antibiotics are applied. Honey, on the other hand, has been found to stop the development of such biofilms. The mechanism is unclear, but may be the result of the fructose and glucose in the honey keeping the biofilm from being able to adhere to the wound tissue.

At the same time, manuka honey has also been shown to reduce the production of tiny anchors called *adhesins* that *Streptococcus pyogenes* — the cause of many infectious diseases, from skin infections to strep throat — needs to start biofilm binding. As a result, there is some suggestion that manuka honey should not just be used to treat established infections in wounds, but should also be included as a preventative.

With *Staphylococcus aureus*, including antibiotic-resistant strains, manuka honey has been shown to eradicate biofilms. Dr Liz Harry and her team at the University of Sydney are doing pioneering work in this regard, and have recently shown that the honey can in some cases penetrate the biofilm and kill embedded cells underneath.* In *E. coli*, a concentration of only 5% manuka honey reduced biofilm amounts by 95%, a concentration 10 times lower than what would be needed to kill the bacteria itself. In this case, reduction in the activity of genes was involved. So there appear to be two processes at work: the sugars in honey, and, in the case of manuka honey, an additional compound as well.

Finally, there is the impact honey has on the virulence of bacteria. These microbes' ability to grow and multiply is beyond phenomenal. In the time it takes your average human cell to divide just once, a single bacterial cell can make as many as 280,000 *billion* copies of itself, provided it has the right conditions and enough food. So, as you can imagine, anything that can slow that process down can greatly affect the bacteria's ability to do enough harm to create what we call a disease.* Manuka honey has been found to affect genes associated with something called *quorum sensing*, a means whereby a bacterial cell assesses the density of others around it, and as a result 'decides' to make some more. One gene involved relates to a bacteria's ability to source the iron it needs to carry out division. In other words, manuka honey has the ability to interfere with the bacteria at the most basic level, how it regulates itself.*

Honey as an antibacterial system

It is said that we live in the golden age of antibiotics, although of course as 'ages' go it hasn't been all that long, with the first man-made antibiotics only coming into general use after World War II. But as we have already discussed, bacteria have a remarkable ability to become resistant to antibiotics. When they can reproduce hundreds of thousands of billions of times per day, it is inevitable that in the process of copying their genes sometimes tiny pieces of chromosomes might get a bit jumbled, and the odd mutation will occur. And when that mutation allows even one bacterial cell to survive the particular mode of destruction that is produced by an often very specific chemical contained in a drug, lots more of that new form of the bacteria will start to multiply and take over.

Scientists are extremely worried about this developing trend, especially since we tend to use some antibiotics so indiscriminately (including feeding them routinely as a 'growth promoter' in farm animals). And in fact recent reviews of the problem have revealed that bacteria are now developing resistance at a faster pace than we are developing new antibiotics to take the place of the ones that no longer work. There are now bacterial species that are resistant to every manufactured antibiotic on the market, and bacteria capable of surviving antiseptics have also emerged.*

So the obvious question to ask is: won't these cunning bacteria develop resistance to manuka honey as well? It is impossible to ever know for sure, of course, but all the signs point to honey being a very special case in this regard. There certainly doesn't seem to be any sort of cross-resistance, at least. Antibiotic-resistant strains of major disease-causing bacteria have been shown to be just as sensitive to manuka honey as non-resistant strains. Bacteria known for their ability to become resistant to antibiotics have also been 'trained' using honey, since developing resistance in these organisms is so easy you can do it in the lab. In one study no signs of resistance were seen, even though the same bacteria started well down that path in response to the use of a synthetic antibiotic.

In another study, conducted by the indefatigable Rose Cooper and her Cardiff team, over time it took higher concentrations of manuka honey to kill the same bacteria, although no mutations of bacteria that would be needed to produce resistance were found. The researchers concluded that, so long as high concentrations of manuka honey with good non-peroxide antibacterial activity were used in clinical practice, the risk of developing resistant bacteria was low.* Interestingly, the reason this may be so has a lot to do with manuka honey being a natural product, rather than the sort of synthetic compound more commonly preferred these days by medical authorities. In those antibiotics, a great deal of effort and money has gone into engineering a particular chemical substance to have a specific effect on bacteria, as for instance breaking down its cell wall. Unfortunately, however, once bacteria mutate their way around that effect, the chemical no longer works.

As we have just seen, however, honey works on multiple targets; so many in fact that it may be difficult if not impossible for bacteria to mutate their way around all of them. It is for this reason that drug makers are now looking at similar types of multi-pronged approaches in the new antibiotics they might create. It would also seem to make sense to use manuka honey together with existing antibiotics to create a synergistic effect. In this case, the honey might knock out the resistant strain of bacteria in an infection, making the antibiotic effective again.

Honey is so effective against bacteria because it is in essence a *system*, and like all such natural systems it has withstood the test of time because it has a number of overlapping elements. The way honey is 'designed' would be quite familiar to systems engineers who work with complicated machines like aircraft. In a plane, if one crucial feature such as a dial or switch doesn't work, there needs to be another feature that can compensate to ensure the survival of those on board. The system has to be robust, not fragile.*

Natural selection is very good at creating robust systems. As we have seen, the body's immune system has any number of components to deal with an infection. If one isn't enough, other components are able to take over. And multiple components are always at work. The same thing is found in plants, and they produce a wide variety of chemicals that can work against the pests that plague them, because of course they can't run away from danger the way animals can. And it is the same with honey. If it were like a synthetic drug and had only one component that attacked a certain feature of a species of bacteria, the microbes would soon develop resistance. Man-made antibiotics are therefore inherently fragile. It is only because of an array of compounds and effects that honey has been able to withstand those sorts of organism over the millennia. If an immune system is a set of biological compounds and processes within an organism that protects against disease, it is not too much of a stretch to think of honey as such a system, a system created by bees.

When it comes to the antibacterial activity of honey, it would appear that a food really can be a better medicine than the ones we humans manufacture ourselves, at least in the long run. That certainly appears to be what the honey bees have found over the past 10 million years or so. If bacteria and fungi had worked out a way to mutate in order to withstand the various ways honey rendered them incapable of using the energy-rich substance as a nutrient, spoilage would have been the inevitable result. And no doubt the bees would have turned to some other less-perishable food source a very long time ago.

A real pain in the stomach

Bill Floyd's press release in 1992 didn't just 'grow legs' because it announced the discovery of non-peroxide activity in manuka honey. It also captured people's attention because it mentioned stomach ulcers. In fact, almost half of the release talked about giving 'the stressed-out executive in fear of a stomach ulcer new hope'.

There were already a number of reports in the science literature about the use of honey in the treatment of stomach disorders, including colitis and gastric ulcers in test animals, and successful treatment of gastritis and peptic ulcers in humans. Most of the case studies came from Eastern Europe and Islamic countries where the traditional use of honey to relieve stomach complaints had carried through to modern medical practice.

There was also a famous clinical study in which honey was used to treat children with gastroenteritis, a significant health problem throughout the developing world. Gastroenteritis can be caused by either bacterial infection or a virus. In either case, the dehydration that results from vomiting and diarrhoea is a significant associated effect that can cause death, especially in infants, since they have a faster metabolism than adults, and their skin surface area compared with their total body weight is larger. The study of 169 infant and child patients in South Africa with bacterial gastroenteritis found that those given honey recovered almost twice as fast as those receiving standard treatment. The honey was found to be as effective as the glucose used in oral rehydration liquids, and its antibacterial activity cleared infections associated with bacterial diarrhoea. The study gave hope to health professionals in the poorest areas of the world that a food product that was both inexpensive and readily available could be a life-saver for infants sick with what we commonly call 'stomach bugs'.*

However, Bill Floyd's press release took those reports one step further. As we mentioned previously, a recent study carried out in Peter Molan's lab had found manuka honey with non-peroxide activity inhibited the growth of a particularly nasty bacterium called *Helicobacter pylori*.

Over 400 bacterial species are present in our stomachs, and without them we wouldn't be able to digest our food. But not all of these bacteria are that benign. And thanks to the pioneering work of two Australian researchers in 1982, who won Nobel Prizes for their efforts, we now know that the cause of most stomach ulcers is usually *H. pylori*. Although half of us have these bacteria in our gastrointestinal system, they only cause symptoms in about 20% of cases. When they do, however, the illness can be very painful and difficult to cure. Use of standard antibiotics is expensive, and relapse verges on 100% after two years, since the drugs do not reduce the inflammation or heal what is in effect a wound of the stomach lining.

Graduate students at the University of Waikato were able to show that all species of bacteria causing gastroenteritis were sensitive to the honey, but that only manuka honey with non-peroxide activity showed inhibition against the *H. pylori*. Complete inhibition occurred at 5% honey concentration.* As a result of these findings, work got under way to set up a clinical trial in New Zealand to study the effect of taking manuka honey orally to reduce the levels of the *H. pylori*. Unfortunately, however, the study was abandoned before completion because of the failure of clinicians to secure enough test subjects. Results did show, however, that patients taking manuka honey with non-peroxide activity reported significant relief of associated symptoms (pain and discomfort) compared with those taking manuka honey without the activity.

Sometime later a very small study of 12 patients with ulcers was carried out in the United Kingdom using a special breath test to confirm whether they had *H. pylori* infections. The patients were given manuka honey with non-peroxide honey equivalent to 12% phenol for a month. However, at the end of that time the test showed that the bacteria were still present. The researchers concluded that if honey was effective in reducing the symptoms of stomach ulcers, it wasn't doing it by eliminating the *H. pylori*.* And that is still pretty much how it stands. In this case, we have a traditional use of honey that clearly relieves the symptoms of stomach complaints. And our science-based inquiry provided a suggestion that maybe something else might be at work as well, since 'test-tube' studies showed manuka honey with its special antibacterial activity was able to kill a bacteria that only recently had been discovered to cause many of the stomach ulcers that produced those symptoms in the first place.

Perhaps this association between manuka honey and *H. pylori* represented a jump in logic, although the jury is still out. Questions still need to be answered, such as what happens to the honey's special activity once it enters the acidity of the stomach. Recent research suggests that *H. pylori* is one of those bacteria that succeeds by forming biofilms, and so interest in manuka honey and the stomach may be renewed since we know it has non-adhesion effects. And certainly the anti-inflammatory abilities of manuka honey in particular may play a significant role in alleviating the pain associated with stomach ulcers. There is obviously much we still have to learn.

One thing is certain, however. There are times when our ability to explain things in medical terms still isn't able to provide all the answers. Human experience is also an important judge. People in China don't need a Western medical authority to tell them whether or not honey is good for the stomach, or explain exactly the components involved. They have been taking it for centuries for indigestion, arguably as long as honey has been used in the West on wounds and burns. Honey is an important component of Chinese medicine, and users have no doubt that it works.

Skincare and jock itch ... why there is honey in your shampoo

If you use a moisturisng lotion for your hands or skin, there is a good chance the product might contain honey. You will also often find honey as an ingredient in shampoos and conditioners, cleansing milks, suncare products and lip ointments.* We tend to think that these products are a fairly recent phenomenon, but the use of honey in skincare and cosmetics goes back in time just as far as its medical applications. Nomadic tribes in the Middle East used honey as an ingredient in cosmetics as long ago as 4500 BC, and the Egyptians added it to the milk in which Cleopatra bathed. Later, the Romans included it as a main ingredient (with olive oil, of course) in a facial pack to improve the skin.

One of the rarest sorts of books, a medieval medical treatise written by a woman (Trotula of Salerno), includes information on the use of honey in skin moisturisers, hair dye, and lip and face treatments. And in the Renaissance, honey was part of the everyday hair and skincare in Italy. In fact, many of the formulas had remained unchanged from Roman times. Honey seemed particularly popular in Venice, where it was mixed with alum and sulphur to create a golden tone in women's hair. The same can be said for the East, where honey has long been a traditional treatment for acne and other facial skin conditions. In Japan, women used it daily to help reduce wrinkles on their hands. It was also used as a traditional face mask preparation in Arab countries, and for the treatment of freckles and white spots in the Indian subcontinent.

Once again, however, modern science can't help but ask the question, what is it in honey that makes it useful in skincare? Claims made for cosmetics aren't subject to the same level of intense scrutiny and clinical evidence-based assessment required for medical drugs, but we still often wonder what the basis is for including honey in a shampoo or a hand cream. Much of it relates to the ways we have already seen honey working to help heal wounds. The antibacterial activity is very important, particularly in relation to breaks in the outer skin layer caused by skin allergies or chapped skin. These breaks aren't in themselves an infection, but once the underlying tissue is exposed it is an attractive place for bacteria to grow.

Skin is also a favourite haunt of another vast group of organisms called fungi. For humans, the world would be a lot less tasty (but perhaps more sober) if it weren't for the yeast-part of the fungal kingdom. But other species of fungi find that humans are a very useful niche (literally) in which to live. As it turns out, manuka honey in particular has been shown in laboratory studies to inhibit the growth of a number of different skin fungi that cause *tinea*, a broad range of skin diseases commonly known by their far more irritating-sounding names, including ringworm, athletes' foot and jock itch, as well as the very unattractive fungal toenail. And tests on *Malassezia* yeasts that are associated with scaly skin, including dandruff, suggest that they are also susceptible to honey. Interestingly, the antifungal property in honey doesn't appear to be caused only by hydrogen peroxide, or even by the osmotic effect of high sugar concentration. Something else is at work as well.*

The other factor, of course, is the encouragement of tissue regrowth that honey provides. This is obvious in a big wound, but just as important in small skin tears, as well as the regeneration of cells just below the harder, protective layer of the skin itself. As time goes on we are beginning to understand the direct cellular processes involved, including the ability of honey to activate several of the communication substances that cells produce. The processes include white blood cells stimulated to dispose of dead tissue, cell markers triggered to repair the growth of new cells, and tissue cells called *keratinocytes* that are induced to transform from one form to another. Keratinocytes make up 90% of the cells in the *epidermis*, the outermost layer of the skin.

Honey as an antioxidant

No discussion of our skin, or any other part of our body, for that matter, would be complete without talking about oxidation. It is a process that, while sometimes damaging to our bodies, is also ironically linked to how we manage to survive at all. None of us can do without oxygen. We breathe it in, blood carries it to our cells, and we put it to work with nutrients from the food we eat to make energy in a process called *metabolism*. Unfortunately, however, oxygen is a highly reactive molecule. In the form called a *free radical* it has a missing electron, and because electrons want to be in pairs, the single electron in the free radical tries to find mates by *breaking down* (reacting with) molecules it comes into contact with. It is this process that makes iron rust, and turns an apple brown. When it happens in our body, it can be very damaging to parts of our cells. Reacting with proteins can keep enzymes from carrying out their many tasks, while damage to DNA can cause mutations, cell death and sometimes even cancer.

As well, the *mitochondria* — the actual energy makers present in our cells — can leak non-radicals like hydrogen peroxide. There are normally enzymes in cells that deal with the damaging effects of these non-radicals by converting them into oxygen and water. Unfortunately, however, the conversion isn't 100% effective, and as a result peroxides persist in the cell. While these products are part of normal cell functioning, excessive amounts can cause serious effects, including degenerative diseases. And the effect can be cumulative, as damage reduces metabolic efficiency, producing more oxidation in a sort of chain reaction.

Where problems can arise is during times of oxidative stress, where levels of *reactive oxygen species* (called ROS) can increase dramatically, causing significant damage to cell structures. What happens is that more ROS are produced during metabolism than the cells are able to render harmless, and the resulting damage is greater than the cells can repair. Cells stop functioning properly, and, in the process we call *ageing*, fewer new cells are produced to take the place of damaged cells. The good news, however, is that dealing with ROS is essential to life, and our bodies have elaborate *antioxidant* systems in place for that purpose. Antioxidants are compounds that scavenge for ROS, prevent their formation, and even repair the damage that they cause. Antioxidants work because they have extra electrons they are able to donate to free radicals. When that happens, ROS no longer seek out an electron from within the cell. Best of all, even though the antioxidant has lost an electron, it doesn't have the need to go out and find one itself from other molecules. It can handle this change in electrons without becoming reactive itself.

Antioxidants are produced within the body, and include enzyme and non-enzyme components in the liver and red blood cells. Cells themselves also have two lines of antioxidant defence, the cellular membrane containing vitamin E, and scavengers inside including vitamin C. Antioxidants can also come into the body from foods such as fruits, vegetables, seeds and nuts. The plants that produce these things have created antioxidants of their own in a wide range of their cells to protect themselves against oxidation, particularly when they suffer oxidative stress from environmental conditions like UV radiation and excess heat.

Honey, it has been discovered, has quite high antioxidant activity relative to other foods, and can intercept free radicals before they can do any damage to the body. This 'pre-emptive' antioxidant activity has been found in some honeys (including especially New Zealand honeydew) to be able to mop up free radicals at levels even better than large doses of vitamin C.

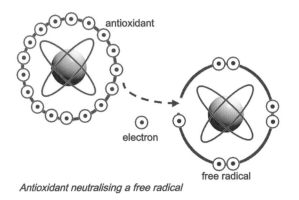

Antioxidant neutralising a free radical

An antioxidant like honey has an extra electron that it can donate to free radicals, nullifying oxygen molecules that can cause human cells to stop functioning properly.

Skin cells are one of the real battle grounds of oxidation. In a wound, those white blood cells that deal to dead tissue cells, as well as to bacteria trying to get inside, produce lots of free radicals as part of their metabolism. This can interfere with the healing process, inactivating important enzymes and proteins needed to coordinate the various cells involved, and even damage DNA. When that happens, the production of *collagens* and other compounds that make up new granulation tissues is disrupted — and these are the very products needed to cover over a wound and grow out new skin.

One of the types of skin damage we all experience from time to time is sunburn. In this case the exposure of our skin to strong and prolonged ultraviolet (UV) radiation creates an immediate effect of skin redness, caused by increased blood flow to the lower layers, and the inflammation effects of the innate immune system. There are also delayed effects, such as premature skin ageing and even cancer. UV radiation penetrates easily through skin. It creates direct damage to DNA in cells, causing them to die. It also damages lower layers by oxidation, creating ROS, which can lead to further damage in cells. So sunburn doesn't just create direct damage to the skin. It creates free radicals as well. This is the reason that antioxidant compounds are put into sunscreens, as well as into skincare lotions and creams.

Honey has always been an ingredient in these sorts of products because of its moisturising properties. It has the ability to both draw moisture from the air and pull moisture from lower down in the body's tissues up towards the surface layer of the skin. Now, however, it is becoming increasingly clear that honey plays an important antioxidant role as well.*

Inflammation and immune stimulation: the cutting edge of honey research

As we saw in the previous chapter, inflammation is one of body's first reactions to both wounds and infections. Damaged cells release chemicals that increase blood flow, and signal those white blood cells to the problem area. Swelling occurs, and with it there is often extreme pain. Inflammation is an important part of the immune system, but because it often produces major discomfort, we use anti-inflammatory drugs to reduce its effects. However, those drugs often have side effects. For instance, they hold back the healing process in wounds and burns, and cannot be used for eye infections.

We seem to have always known that honey reduces inflammation, which is the reason why many cultures have used it to help alleviate the pain and swelling associated with a sore throat. More recently, that ability has been tested in a clinical setting, with trials conducted on patients with conditions or undergoing treatments that are known to create significant inflammatory effects. The most important of these trials, and the one that really helps improve the lives of people suffering painful side effects, is the use of honey to reduce the inflammation caused by radiation therapy. At least four clinical studies have been carried out on people receiving radiotherapy for head and neck cancer. In each case, the group of patients that were given honey to hold in their mouth during treatment experienced less pain, swelling and ulcers in the soft tissues of the mouth, tongue and throat compared with those not using the honey.

Another type of pain and inflammation many of us have experienced as children occurs when tonsils are removed. In a clinical study, the lucky group of children who were given honey every hour, rather than a saline solution control, asked for less paracetamol, a sure sign that they were feeling less pain. As someone with a sense of humour pointed out, however, the study did mean that a teaspoon of honey made less of the medicine go down!

A trial was also conducted comparing a manuka honey lozenge with sugarless chewing gum. After three weeks, patients who sucked on the honey product had significantly less bleeding and inflammation of the gums. Another clinical study produced a similar result when comparing manuka honey added to mouthwash with the same sort of sugar-free gum. Part of the effect may be caused by manuka honey's ability to keep the biofilm of nasty mouth bacteria from adhering to the teeth at the gum line. But there appears to be an anti-inflammatory component involved as well.

From these and other studies it is clear that we know a lot more about how honey affects patients with various kinds of inflammation than we do about the actual substances and mechanisms involved. The antioxidant effect of honey certainly seems to play a role, since oxidation is a significant component associated with inflammation. But there is bound to be more to it than just that.

What we do know is that manuka honey has a more pronounced anti-inflammatory effect than other honeys, and recently Amanda Bean, a PhD student at Peter Molan's lab, identified a protein that bees add to honey called *apalbumin-1*. Obviously it is a hard substance to identify, since it should be present in all honey that bees make, no matter what the floral source. Amanda, however, was able to show that the same special ingredient found in manuka honey that causes its non-peroxide activity reacts with this protein, and makes the honey much more anti-inflammatory.*

All the books say that the body's response to wounds is highly complex, and that certainly seems to carry over to the immune-system effects of honey. While on the one hand it contains anti-inflammatory components, we also know that it stimulates parts of that system, including those cell communicators (called *cytokines*) that stimulate white blood cells, as well as those molecules called growth factors that trigger tissue cells to fill in and close over wounds. This *immuno-stimulatory* effect of honey helps to explain why honey can help in the healing of persistent wounds where the body for some reason doesn't repair itself as well as it should. Honey seems to be able to provide a 'jump-start' for the immune system in this regard. Determining exactly what components in honey produce this immune-stimulation effect is at the cutting edge of honey research. One of the compounds seems to be another protein bees add that is the same as that found in the royal jelly that the nurse bees feed the queen and young larvae. Another is a compound called *arabinogalactan*, two single molecule sugars (arabinose and galactose) attached to a protein. Arabinogalactans are found in many plants, and are known to stimulate the immune system. Recently a research group at the University of Auckland isolated a particular arabinogalactan from kanuka honey, and showed that the immune stimulation activity of different honeys depends on the amount of this compound.*

Natural products and modern medicine: honey as a test case

There are many more therapeutic properties and medical uses for honey.* For instance, it contains oligosaccharides that are *prebiotics*, meaning that they stimulate the growth and activity of beneficial bacteria in the human digestive system. Clinical trials show that it can also be effective in the treatment of eye infections, a use that goes back to ancient times. And honey — in particular manuka honey with non-peroxide antibacterial activity — has an anti-fungal effect on *Candida*, the cause of thrush. Recently honey and yoghurt were trialled successfully as a means of controlling this painful infection in pregnant women.*

Manuka honey has even been shown to kill the seven species of bacteria most commonly found in mastitis in dairy cows. As a result, it is now an ingredient in one of the leading brands of teat sanitisers in New Zealand. The honey protects the teats from becoming cracked and chaffed, as well as helping keep infections at bay. It is a somewhat ironic use, however, because, back when beekeepers had a hard time finding a sale for manuka honey, it was sometimes added to supplemental feed the cows were given to improve the ration's taste.*

The potential obviously exists to create a range of health-related products containing honey. However, it takes a great deal of time and money to get the sort of meta-analysis that government regulators demand before a therapeutic claim can be put on the label. As a result, you are not likely to find many such products on your pharmacy shelf anytime soon. Manuka honey, though, is the exception. The acceptance of manuka honey in woundcare, including by that most exacting of medical registration authorities, the FDA, is truly significant. In fact, it represents something of a test case as far as natural products are concerned. Honey is a natural substance that hasn't been cut up into individual ingredients, synthesised by industrial chemists, put through the patent-clinical trials-medical registration process, and then offered as a 'better living through chemistry' wonder drug. To have it accepted by the medical establishment would seem to be almost unprecedented in this day and age.

As Ralf Schlothauer — an Adjunct Associate Professor with the Food Science Programme at the University of Auckland, and someone closely involved with the latest research on the therapeutic properties of manuka — has pointed out, honey has at least six individual antibacterial components, four anti-inflammatory, and two immuno-stimulatory ones. If it were an industrially produced drug, with even three of those components, like the standard three-antibiotic treatment for *H. pylori*, to obtain certification for it, a drug company would not only have to do the efficacy and safety tests on each of those components individually, it would also have to do the same with each of the combinations. For three drugs, there are six combinations. The costs are extremely high to do something like that. With honey, which has a total of at least 12 components, that makes almost half a billion combinations. According to Ralf, 'That's why natural compounds like honey can never be excluded from modern medical consideration. To make a drug like that and get it approved through the normal processes would be impossible.'

And if you delve into the matter, you find that natural products are very important to medical science. As Bill Bryson points out in his wonderful book *A Short History of Nearly Everything*, only 1% of flowering plants have ever been tested for their medicinal properties. But the ones that have are responsible for providing us with the source of fully one quarter (25%) of all our modern prescribed medicines, and they come from a total of only 40 plants. Another 16% come from animals or microbes. As he also points out, plants are a very efficient way of discovering useful medical compounds. They have already gone through countless generations of trial and error, sorting out what works against things like bacteria and fungi and viruses.

A big reason natural products have given us so many ideas for medicines is quite simply that we have been able to see that they work. Finding out how they work is a taller order, as we have seen, but you don't need that depth of understanding to create a remedy that has a useful effect. And certainly going in the other direction has proven to be a lot harder.

As Bryson says, when chemists try to create useful substances 'from scratch' in the lab, they use a method called *combinatorial chemistry* that can generate up to 40,000 compounds at a time. But the results are totally random, and almost always useless. Those sorts of 'un-natural' compounds can also end up having dangerous side effects, ones that unfortunately don't always show up right away.* With natural products, on the other hand, there is a huge natural laboratory, often filled with all sorts of plant and bug and animal 'guinea pigs'. No ethics committee approval was required. And because over countless generations we have become expert in passing down the 'folk knowledge' of what works, and what should be avoided, along with observing how all the other creatures around us have reacted to the same things, we already have a good idea about natural product safety and efficacy. When you synthesise a drug without any natural background, on the other hand, you're back to square one.

In modern times, however, what has happened is that pharmaceutical companies have figured out the active compounds in these natural products, and then synthesised them. Some people think this is some sort of great industrial conspiracy, but in fact because of the regulatory requirements involved, and the large-scale clinical trials that evidence-based assessment demands, it often takes a molecule that can be synthesised and patented to generate the down-stream sales needed to fund the up-stream work. The result, though, is that we now have a medical system that believes in the superiority of synthetic drugs. The author Michael Pollan even argues that the prejudice towards manufactured medicines and away from natural ones comes from the cultural bias the Church needed to create, as it became a widespread European institution, in order to woo the common people away from paganism (literally the worshipping of nature).*

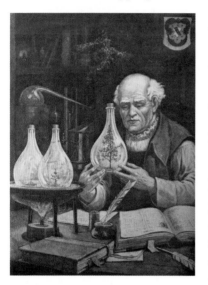

Paracelsus, the father of pharmacology, who was able to put 'pagan' learning about natural products into a form acceptable to the Church.

That point can certainly be argued, but what we do know is that medical chemistry (called *pharmacology*) had its beginnings with people who studied nature so intently, and believed so much in its power, that they made up potions containing highly potent plants, animals and their extracts. Unfortunately we still call such people by the derogatory name 'witch doctors'. Indeed, the sixteenth-century originator of pharmacology, Paracelsus, who invented amongst much else the drug laudanum, a natural product in the form of an opium extract that became the most important pharmaceutical drug for the next 400 years, said he learned about chemistry (or alchemy) and the making of medicines from such 'old wives, gipsies and sorcerers'. Part of Paracelsus's genius, however, was putting this pagan learning into a form that was acceptable to the Church-controlled powers that be.

Pollan's theory might help explain why we have this dualism and often antipathy in the West to remedies that are deemed to be 'alternative' because they happen to be natural, a dualism that does not exist in the East. It is a dualism that is neatly defined by the two contrasting messages Hippocrates gave us: the power of observation and investigation, and the instruction to 'let food be thy medicine'. Practitioners of mainstream Western medicine are likely to argue that the dualism exists because their drugs are more sophisticated, technological and science-based. There can be no denying the truth in that statement. The point is simply that we shouldn't believe too much in the superiority of our modern chemistry to synthesise drugs 'out of the blue'. When we do that we aren't being honest about where we got the idea for many of those chemical compounds from in the first place. To extol the virtues of natural products like honey certainly isn't to denigrate the wondrous achievements of modern medicine and pharmaceutical science. It is more a matter of giving both sides of the divide we have created, at least in West, their due.

It is hard to know where this argument will go in the future. But there is one demand from the world's regulators of medicines that every natural product sold for therapeutic purposes must face. One of pharmacology's great contributions has been the realisation that medicines of whatever type must be standardised. We need to be able to measure the effect of the product, using the most objective means possible, and identify the amount of the active ingredients it contains. It is the *quid pro quo* argument — if natural products are going to be used in modern medicine, they need to be processed to the same standards of hygiene and testing as any other pharmaceutical. And customers need to have absolute assurance that they are getting what it says on the label. For honey, and particularly for manuka honey, that turns out to be not quite as simple as it might seem.

Eight

ONE FROM
ANOTHER

Beekeepers need to prepare themselves for questions. Because, let's face it, first and foremost they are a novelty. They represent a tiny minority, not just in the community, but in the world at large. Very few people keep honey bees, for a good reason — they sting. And most of us have a strong and very sensible fear of bees that is difficult if not impossible to overcome. At the same time, however, we find bees fascinating creatures, especially now that they have become 'poster insects' for environmental sustainability. They are a sort of 'canary in the coal mine' for worries about our ability to exist for very much longer on the planet.

The problem is that we just can't get our heads around putting on a veil, using a smoker, and diving into a bunch of boxes throbbing with insects that even individually can cause such pain. People who can do that must be wired differently from the rest of us. So when we meet a beekeeper we pump them with questions, and the questions are usually the same. Along with 'How did you get into beekeeping?', 'Are honey bees really disappearing?', and the inevitable 'Does it hurt when you get stung?', the one question that is most difficult to answer is, 'How do you tell one honey from another?' For anyone who has been a beekeeper for any amount of time, and especially for any commercial beekeeper, the answer to that last question is very difficult to put into words. It is something they just know. The taste is imprinted on their tongue (and their brain) as precisely as wine types are for sommeliers. They also know a honey's colour, its smell, and even sometimes its special physical characteristics.

If they are really dedicated beekeepers, and move their hives from place to place to increase production during a season that can extend from late spring through to early autumn, they are also pretty good botanists. They may not be able to spout genus and species, but they certainly know the common names of honey sources, along with their bloom periods.

Almost all flowering plants have a specific time of the year when they bloom intensively, and when the nectar is produced in greatest profusion. The duration of these *honey flows* is usually only about three or four weeks, and beekeepers learn quite quickly where the best stands of these plants are located, particularly if they are wild species. They find places to put their beehives that are as near to such locations as possible, and they jealously guard these apiaries from other beekeepers. Some beekeepers may even know the colour of the pollen that the nectar-producing flowers produce. The reason, of course, is that they see the pollen being brought back to the hive in big, round loads, packed onto the hind legs of the foraging worker bees.

Having this sort of knowledge is one thing. But to be able to explain it all to a non-beekeeper in a sentence or two, especially before they get the sense that they are boring the listener, is very difficult. And as it turns out, it is also not that easy trying to explain it to customers, or the regulatory authorities whose job it might be to protect the public's right to know the source of their food.

Part of the problem is that honey produced in bulk quantities from a single floral source only happens under very rare circumstances. One example might be *canola*, the more user-friendly Canadian-derived name for oil seed rape. In the western prairie areas of that country, farmers sometimes plant vast, half-mile by half-mile *quarter sections* of the plant, and when it blooms the attractiveness of the nectar and the density of the bloom, along with a lack of nearby competing sources of either planted crops or weeds, means that sometimes hives will produce pure canola honey. This is especially the case if the honey crop is removed by the beekeeper before the canola has finished flowering and any other sources that might be a further bee-flight distance away start to produce nectar.

Another example can be found in New Zealand. Rangitoto Island is a volcanic cone that sits in the middle of the Hauraki

Gulf, just off of Auckland. It was formed by a series of eruptions only 550–600 years ago, and can sometimes look almost black from the mainland, since of course it is mostly composed of dark lava rock. Everyone knows Rangitoto's distinctive conical shape, but very few realise that it is host to the largest pohutukawa forest in the world. So when the distinctive bright-red flowers bloom around Christmas time, several barge-loads of beehives are brought to the island.* But even here, on an island far enough away from the mainland that the bees aren't likely to fly across to get much pollen and nectar from other blooming plants, you can't be absolutely sure that the honey produced from those hives is 100% pure pohutukawa. There are over 200 species of plant on the island, and while none of them are as widely spread, or produce as much nectar as the big pohutukawa trees, you can never guarantee that the bees didn't find at least a few other blooming plants to visit as well.

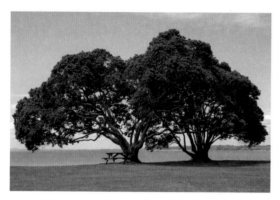

The pohutukawa tree with its distinctive bright red flowers. These trees cover Rangitoto Island, and provide honey bees with the nectar they turn into single-source pohutukawa honey.

That's the thing with honey bees. They are some of the world's foremost collectors. They intensely fly all over an area of at least 3 kilometres in radius, and if a flower has either pollen or honey or both, chances are that flower will receive at least one visit from a bee, especially if the area is being searched over by 20,000 or more foragers per hive, and there are 20 or 30 hives in the apiary. It is for this reason that the *Codex Alimentarius* (Latin for 'Book of Food'), the set of recommended food standards developed by the Food and Agriculture Organisation of the United Nations, says that honey may be called a single floral source if it 'comes wholly or *mainly* from that particular source'.

Colour, flavour and physico-chemistry

Beekeepers have always known the taste and colour of different honeys, and for a long time that has also been the primary means by which honey processers and packers have differentiated one honey from another. When the honey in question is a widely produced one, such as clover, and fetches what can sometimes be a commodity-type price, getting it right perhaps isn't quite so important. If it looks like what we think of as clover honey, or even just pasture honey, and it doesn't have a distinctively different taste, no one is likely to object. If, on the other hand, the honey is much rarer, and sought after by discerning buyers, it is far more important that it should conform to the memory the customer has of the same honey they purchased previously. Beekeepers aren't the only ones who become quite discerning in their ability to identify honey from different sources. Lovers of honey who are the end-users of the product get to know one honey from another as well.

This is the reason the Honey Marketing Authority (HMA) in New Zealand employed honey graders. They were independent professionals whose job it was to determine whether a honey was mainly from one floral source or another. Just as importantly, they also provided an assurance to the big honey buyers in Europe regarding the quality of the honey contained in the barrels the authority exported.

The main criteria the graders used was colour, since back then it was the number-one criterion used internationally, especially for commodity-type honeys that competed on the world market with similar honeys produced in other countries. The colour-determining device they used was called a *Pfund grader*, a simple machine that contained a glass cell for holding the liquid honey, and a wedge of amber-coloured glass. Turning a small knob moved the wedge along the edge of a ruler; the further it went along the wedge, the darker the colour. When the colour of the wedge and the honey matched, the distance along the ruler, expressed in millimetres, became the objective means of identifying how dark or light the honey was.

Other types of comparator devices have since been developed, including glass bottles filled with liquid of different shades and *turbidity* (the amount of light that can pass through), and the Lovibond Honey Grader, which looks very much like those

Viewmasters that kids used to peer through in the 1950s. But the net result is the same. Either the honey is given a millimetre grade, or described using a standardised phrase — from *water-white* to *dark amber*, with various steps in between.

The problem with colour is that honey from a particular floral source can vary considerably in colour, depending on plant varieties, soil type, and even climatic conditions. Manuka honey is a good case in point. The honey has a wide range of shades, which also appears to depend on where in the country it is produced. It has been said that beekeepers in the South Island invariably produce a much lighter manuka honey than their counterparts in the North Island. And an important source of information on world honey sources lists the honey as falling in a wide range of between 69 mm and 140 mm on the Pfund scale.*

In the days of the HMA, the lighter the colour of a commodity-type honey, the higher the price it could command on the international market. That is still often the case today. Off-tastes can be important, especially with the lighter-coloured and generally milder-tasting honeys. But it is only with high-value honeys that floral source is really essential, and that is where the skill of the honey grader can come to the fore. A honey grader needs a trained palette, and reference samples to compare flavours. Flavour is also something that can quickly tire the taste buds, or at least affect our brain's ability to make the subtle distinctions in a food that is always predominantly sweet. It is not a job where you can really push yourself, and there might even be a work hazard involved. Two New Zealand honey graders had to quit their posts because they eventually developed type II diabetes.

The flavour of honey, and to a lesser extent its aroma, is probably honey's most defining attribute, and yet we know very little about what chemicals are involved. Over 500 different volatile compounds have been recorded so far in the various honeys from around the world. And, as any beekeeper will tell you, the strength in the aroma of 'fresh' honey dissipates over time, as it does if the honey has been subjected to a great deal of heating during processing. The flavour of a honey also changes as it ages.

Honey is said to be comprised of *sweet*, *sour* and *bitter* tastes. (Pohutukawa honey produced from trees right along the New Zealand coast is said to taste slightly of *salt* as well.) The two main sugars in honey are glucose and fructose, and the ratio of one to the other doesn't just determine if it will granulate quickly (if it is high in glucose), it also affects how it will taste. If you have ever compared a fizzy drink sweetened with high fructose corn syrup to an energy drink loaded with glucose, you will know that fructose is much sweeter than glucose (by a factor of 2.5 to 1). So a honey high in fructose, such as clover, will taste sweeter than one high in glucose (for instance, pohutukawa). Honeys also vary according to their acidity, and a more acid honey type will have a more bitter taste.

The biggest problem with identifying a honey source using flavour, however, is trying to determine just how 'single-source' the honey really is. If small amounts of a strong-tasting honey are added to a mildly flavoured one, even a panel of experts will declare it to be a blend. However, large amounts of the mild honey can be added to a flavoursome one and those same experts are likely to still call it a single floral source.*

As a result of these issues, chemists have done a lot work on the *physico-chemical* characteristics of various honeys.* By physico-chemical we mean the measurement of obvious physical properties, as well as basic chemical analysis. For instance, different honey types have been found to conduct an electrical current at different rates. Depending on the ratio of fructose to glucose, they also respond differently to polarised light.

As far as the chemistry goes, we already know that different honeys have different levels of acidity. And a special chemical called *hydroxymethylfurfural* (thankfully referred to routinely as HMF) can be measured to determine whether honey has been over-heated to the point that damage has occurred.

There is also thixotropy, that gel-like property that makes manuka honey so hard to extract. Chemists are able to measure the *viscosity* of honey; in other words, how well it flows. But manuka isn't the only honey that is thixotropic. And as an experiment many years ago showed, you can transfer this gel formation from a thixotropic to a non-thixotropic honey like clover merely by transferring the gel-creating protein.*

Perhaps most importantly, however, whatever type of sensory or physical analysis you might make of a certain honey, the fact remains that your assessment is always one step removed from the plants the bees visit to collect the nectar they turn into that honey. It is for this reason that another technique was developed, one that, believe it or not, owes a lot to digging around in ancient kitchens, as well as much older layers of soil.

The problem with pollen

Shapes in the microscopic world can sometimes seem almost unbelievable, and that is certainly the case when it comes to the pollen grains that flowering plants produce. In fact, if we could enlarge those grains to the size of buildings, they would put Walt Disney's Tomorrowland, or even Buckminster Fuller's geodesic domes to shame.

Pollen grains are highly distinctive. In some plant species they are shaped like diamonds and triangles, while others are perfectly round spheres. And the surface of the grain itself can be covered with knobs, grains, rods or clubs. Pollen from the thistle has lots of spiny points sticking out of it, whereas that of the plantain looks like a moon from some distant planet, with little circles that almost seem to be craters caused by miniature asteroids. Some pollen grains are very small, while others can easily be seen with the naked eye. Manuka pollen is finely grained at around 7 microns. It takes 800 grains of this pollen to have the same volume as one grain of nodding thistle pollen.

Pollen grains are nutritional powerhouses, and the little circles are membrane-covered portholes where the pollen tubule carrying the male genetic material bursts out once the grain has been deposited on the flower's stamen. It's then a race against time as the cell grows down the long style and fertilises the flower's ovary before the food energy packed into the pollen grain is used up. The growth rate is amazing, at up to 35 millimetres per hour (the width of slide film). In maize, this single cell can end up being 450 millimetres long (or just under 18 inches).

It is the protein, vitamins and minerals in the nutritional component of pollen grains that make them so useful and attractive to honey bees. They are the only source of these nutrients that are essential for the bees to raise their brood and feed the queen.

But of course honey bees aren't completely efficient in combing pollen off their hairy bodies, packing it into those brightly coloured pellets on their back legs, and bringing them back to their hive. A portion of the grains get into the nectar, and end up in the honey the bees make. So it seemed logical to scientists that if you collected pollen grains from individual plant species, and then compared them with what you found in a sample of honey, that would tell you what plants were involved.

They already had a well-established set of procedures they could use, and even extensive samples of pollen grains to draw on, from a discipline called *palynology* (Greek for 'the study of particles that are strewn'). The analysis of pollen grains found in the excavation of ancient sites has long been used by archaeologists as a means of identifying the sorts of plant species that our ancestors might have utilised. And as we saw previously, botanists used the finding of manuka pollen in soil layers to provide us with an idea of not just how widespread the plant was before the coming of humans to New Zealand, but also where manuka's *Leptospermum* ancestors originated in Australia before the continent became mostly arid.

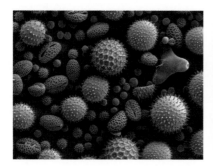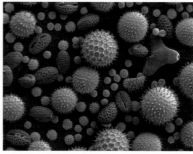

The amazing shapes (and colours) of pollen grains from different plant species. The greyscale version was made using an electron microscope, and the coloured version was then computer-generated to approximate the colours normally associated with each species.

So, beginning in the 1930s, honey analysts began to develop the techniques needed to identify species of pollen grains in honey.* The procedure was fairly simple. It involved taking a given quantity of honey, centrifuging it to get all the pollen into a sludge at the bottom of a test tube, then diluting it again and putting it under the sort of blood cell counter normally used in hospital labs. The practice, called *melissopalynology* (*melisso* = honey) is still in widespread use today. However, it certainly isn't without its problems. As Anna Maurizio, a world expert on melissopalynology has pointed out, the number of pollen grains that get into a volume of honey depends on a range of factors, including the abundance of anthers and pollen, and the floral biology of the plant species, rather than just the amount of nectar produced. As for the honey itself, much depends on the water content of the nectar, the distance the floral sources are from the hive, and beekeeping practices.*

As it turns out, manuka honey provides a prime example of the technique's complexities. Early research suggested that a 'unifloral' sample of manuka honey should have 70% manuka pollen, even though honey produced in New Zealand was deemed to be clover if it only had 45% clover pollen. That seemed counter-intuitive, since honey bees aren't known to collect even small amounts of manuka pollen to bring back to their colonies as food.

There was also the case of a sample of manuka honey with high non-peroxide activity that was determined to only have 15% manuka pollen. Jonathan Stephens and Peter Molan followed up on this case later, and found that even when they collected manuka honey from areas where manuka plants were extensively in bloom, four of the six samples didn't have 70% manuka pollen, including the two samples with the highest non-peroxide activity (17.5 and 15.5 phenol concentration equivalent). The problem was the size of the manuka pollen grains themselves. A percentage of total pollen grains found in the honey wasn't enough, since it took a lot of manuka pollen to make up the same volume as far lesser amounts of other pollens. And it was even the case that pollen could show up in the sample from plants that weren't even blooming at the time the manuka nectar was collected by the bees.* In this case, the culprit was those honey prickers that allowed beekeepers to extract the thixotropic manuka honey from the comb. The pricker doesn't discriminate. Its needles loosen every single cell, and if those cells happened to contain pollen loads that the bees had collected from the flowers of other species previously, that pollen also ended up in the mix. The solution to the problem was to ensure there were over 200,000 grains of manuka pollen in a 10-gram honey sample. In that case the sample could be counted on to be predominately manuka, even if

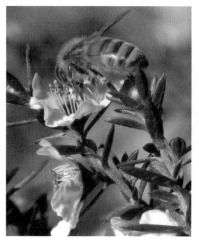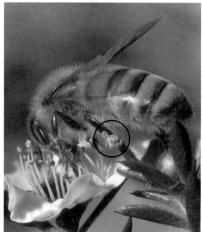

A rare sight – a honey bee with at least a small amount of manuka pollen on its legs.

large amounts of other pollens meant that the honey had far less than 70% manuka pollen.

The most serious issue, however, is that manuka pollen and kanuka pollen look alike. Joy Thompson may have decided that kanuka was in a completely different genus (*Kunzea*), but not even New Zealand's foremost pollen expert could tell pollen grains from the two species apart.*

The problems with pollen content analysis — problems that certainly aren't restricted to manuka — are part of the reason that in Europe, according to a leading authority on honey, 'Pollen content is now regarded as a side method, beside sensory and physico-chemical analysis.'*

Identifying a honey using the standards and techniques that have been developed in Europe, the centre of the 'old world' trade in honey, is difficult to say the least. As a report from the International Honey Commission points out, 'there are no references of natural pure unifloral honeys, as bees always forage on different flower species, even if one species predominates; moreover, it is difficult to identify precisely the discrimination point between multifloral and unifloral honeys, and no analysis allows determining the exact percentage of a given nectar in honey.'*

One thing is certain, however. The $140-million-a-year manuka honey industry wasn't built on how much manuka pollen was present in that honey, no matter what percentage may have been claimed, or whether or not there were problems with under-representation of that pollen. It also isn't sought after for its sensory or physico-chemical characteristics. People have purchased it instead, at prices never before seen for honey, because it has a unique ability to kill disease-causing bacteria, and treat wounds and burns. That sort of consumer recognition falls completely outside the narrow field of vision of honey characterisation, one developed for traditional uses like putting honey on toast. As a result, those old methods of analysis don't really apply.

Manuka honey isn't being sold as a honey. It is being sold as a *nutraceutical*, a food that is also a medicine, and it needs to be judged by new methods that are far more appropriate to its end-use. The guarantee of its antibacterial activity is what pharmaceutical standards require as well.

The magic ingredient revealed

'After finding out manuka honey had a special sort of antibacterial activity, I spent about 20 years trying to find out **what** it was that was responsible for that. ...Then a group working in Dresden, Germany, headed by Professor Thomas Henle, found it when they weren't actually looking for it.' — Peter Molan, 2013

If you have been wondering throughout this book just what the special compound was in manuka honey that gave it a non-peroxide activity not found in other honeys, you can see from this quote that you are in good company. Once manuka honey began to hit the headlines in the 1990s, scientists in various parts of the world began looking for the 'magic ingredient', and, according to Peter, 'There were some big multi-national pharmaceutical companies that tried to do the same. And we all failed.'*

That didn't stop the honey from being sold for its special properties, nor for work to be undertaken to show that it was very effective in treating burns and wounds that didn't heal. As we have seen, there is nothing unusual about that, particularly when the product or treatment has a long-standing history of effectiveness. And being the equivalent of the CSI in our crime novel analogy requires painstaking work. It can take years, using sophisticated and ultra-sensitive chemical analysis machinery, to find the actual cause of the antibacterial activity.

However, beekeepers producing manuka honey, as well as some of the companies marketing it, were concerned about giving some guarantee about its non-peroxide activity. Peter certainly reinforced that point in his articles and lectures. He was worried that manuka honey without good non-peroxide activity might be used in a clinical situation and not produce the proper result. As we have seen, that concern led to the formation of the Active Manuka Honey Association (now called the Unique Manuka Factor Honey Association) that trademarked the Unique Manuka Factor name (UMF™). The rating it used couldn't be more straightforward. It simply involved the plating out of batch samples of the honey, seeing how the honey inhibited the growth of *S. aureus* bacteria, and then comparing the *ring of inhibition* with phenol. The rating was a direct reference back to the concentration of phenol (5+ was equivalent to 5% phenol, 10+ was 10%, etc.).

The test did have its problems, though. Private testing laboratories took over the work that Peter's team was doing in the early days, and there appeared to be differences in some of the results. There are always discrepancies between testing labs, no matter what the test, which is the reason they often carry out *ring trials*, sending the same sample to different labs and comparing measurements. The tests might be 'standard', but there can be at least a bit of an art in carrying them out. There was also sometimes a problem with measuring the 'grey areas' at the edges of the zone of inhibition. And any variations in growing conditions, including temperature and agar gel media, could produce differences. The size of the growth ring itself also isn't directly proportional, since the larger the width of the ring, the bigger the diameter.

Many of these issues have now been resolved, particularly by testing the honey against another honey with a known activity level, so any variations will have the same effect on both samples. As well, multiple tests on a plate are carried out to reduce measuring inconsistencies.*

However, while testing the honey against bacteria provided a direct assessment of at least one of its therapeutic abilities, modern medicine (and in particular pharmaceutical regulatory authorities) always want standardisation, and if possible a measurement of the amount of the active ingredient. So when the team from Dresden Technical University announced in 2008 that they had found the compound, everyone even remotely involved with manuka honey around the world was intensely interested.

Thomas Henle and his colleagues are experts in the field of sugar degradation, which has some less than pleasant effects like spoilage, and some more tasty ones produced by something called the *Maillard reaction*. You may never have heard of this reaction between an amino acid and a sugar, but you certainly know all about the result. It is what puts the dark colour in the outside crust of a loaf of bread, creates the browning in steak, and makes delicious caramel. One of the by-products of the Maillard reaction is a compound called *methylglyoxal*, commonly known as MGO. The compound had previously been found in wine, beer and butter, and in 2004 the Dresden team found it in honey. The levels were quite low, and it in fact may have been the result of excess heating of the product by some packers. However, the group later looked specifically at six samples of manuka honey, and found MGO levels up to 100 times greater than in the previous honeys tested, and higher than in any other food item previously studied. So they decided to test the obvious hypothesis. Sure enough, by using the gel-diffusion assay technique, they showed that the MGO was causing bacterial inhibition broadly similar to the inhibition caused by the honey samples themselves. And what was really amazing was that the MGO in the honey wasn't being produced by the Maillard reaction.*

The rush was now on to conduct research in two areas. Christopher Adams and his colleagues at Waikato University looked at a much larger number of samples of both manuka and non-manuka honeys, confirmed the presence of high levels of MGO, and produced a graph comparing the amount of MGO in a manuka honey sample with the level of bacterial inhibition of the honey measured in percentage of phenol, using the plating technique.* Henle's team produced a similar result, and Henle was confident enough of the findings to say that when present in higher levels, it was directly responsible for 90–95% of manuka honey's special antibacterial activity.[†]

Work also needed to be carried out on MGO in manuka honey to see whether it was safe to consume. MGO isn't found only in foods; it is also a by-product of metabolism, including especially the way cells convert glucose into energy. The body has ways of breaking down MGO produced in this way, but there is a suggestion that the compound might potentially degrade into something called AGE, or *advanced glycation end-products*, that seem to be linked to some diseases, and in particular diabetes where patients have elevated glucose levels in their blood.

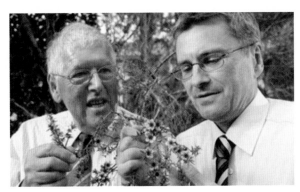

Dr Peter Molan, the discoverer of the special antibacterial activity of manuka honey, and Dr Thomas Henle, who led the team that 26 years later found the major compound responsible for that activity.

So a study was undertaken in New Zealand in 2009 using human volunteers. They were given just over a tablespoon of manuka honey with very high non-peroxide activity (20+) daily for two weeks. The amount of MGO in the honey was approximately 800 milligrams per kilogram. Another group received pasture

---

† As it turned out, there was another component that provided antibacterial activity as well. In an elegant set of experiments conducted in Holland in 2010, manuka honey was 'deconstructed', with the various known antibacterial agents, such as osmolality, hydrogen peroxide and MGO, neutralised in their turn. The researchers found that there was still an antibacterial compound present, a protein added by honey bees called *bee defensin-1*, which had previously been found in royal jelly. Just like the other enzymes, glucose oxidase (which gives honey its acidity, and produces hydrogen peroxide when it is diluted) and invertase (which 'pre-digests' sucrose in nectar, turning it into glucose and fructose), bee defensin-1 is produced in worker bees' hypopharengeal glands, and comes out in the saliva. It is a substance honey bees add to both honey and royal jelly to protect against spoilage, which just goes to show we are still finding out the finer details of the bees' food-preservation recipes. Without a doubt, 'bee spit' is very powerful indeed!

honey. Then they stopped eating the honey for two weeks, and swapped over. Blood and faecal samples were taken weekly by the researchers. The results showed that a well-known AGE by-product of MGO called CML didn't increase in the blood of the volunteers, and nor did an important molecule associated with allergic reactions. At the same time, there was no change to bacteria in the lower gut, suggesting perhaps that manuka honey's effect on indigestion may in fact have been an anti-inflammatory one, rather than antibacterial. The study's authors concluded that consuming manuka honey with 20+ non-peroxide activity was, to quote them, 'safe for healthy individuals'.*

More recently, Thomas Henle and his group have been able to shed more light on the process. The MGO from the honey becomes available in the stomach, and can in fact kill bacteria there such as *Helicobacter pylori*. But the MGO and the honey only remain in the stomach for several hours, and once they move through to the small intestine the pH changes.

As we all know, our stomach produces a lot of acid to help prepare the food we eat for absorption once it passes into the small intestine. And MGO is stable in acidic conditions. However, the Dresden group found that MGO breaks down very quickly once that acid is neutralised in the lower gut. As a result, MGO doesn't find its way into the bloodstream, nor is it found in urine. In wound treatment conditions, it is also likely to be broken down by the higher pH of the blood serum.*

A remarkable discovery

There was still something important to discover, however. How did MGO get into manuka honey in the first place? Samples of nectar taken directly from manuka flowers had little or no MGO, while testing an old sample of manuka honey (which Peter Molan said was 'a positive benefit of not tidying my office') revealed that its non-peroxide antibacterial activity had gone from 12 to over 30. That suggested that MGO was accumulating over time in the honey.

There were rumours that beekeepers were heating their honey to increase its non-peroxide activity, but Henle and his group had already shown that MGO wasn't being produced in manuka honey by the Maillard reaction that occurs when sugars react with proteins in cooking. So something else was clearly involved.

The scene now shifted back to New Zealand. Researchers at the University of Waikato had a look at manuka honey using a very sensitive machine called a *high-performance liquid chromatograph* (better known as HPLC). The device separates substances into individual components, giving a reading like peaks on a graph. And when they looked at MGO, they found another peak right next to it. They compared the amounts of this compound with the non-peroxide antibacterial activity of the honey samples, and while it wasn't as good a fit as with MGO, it still looked promising. So they did some more fancy chemistry, and with the help of another machine that did *nuclear magnetic resonance spectroscopy*, they were able to work out its molecular structure. It was something called *dihydroxyacetone* (or DHA).

When they looked for DHA in manuka nectar they found it in abundance. And when they scraped samples of manuka honey from the comb just after it had been brought in by the bees, while it was still in the process of being ripened, there were low levels of MGO, but high levels of DHA. Then they put that fresh honey in an incubator at hive temperature for several months and looked at it again. The amount of DHA had gone down, while the MGO had gone up.*

DHA, it turned out, was already known by chemists. It is a type of sugar molecule, and is present in aged wine, amongst other foods. When it is in an acid environment, it changes its structure, giving up the elements of water, and turning into MGO. So it was the acidity of honey, produced by the glucose oxidase enzyme that the bees added to nectar (the same one that produces hydrogen peroxide when the honey is diluted), that was setting off the transformation. It was one compound coming from another, and it was all a matter of that 'cooking' the bees do so well.†

---

† One of the side-benefits of the DHA discovery is only now coming to light. Analytical chemists developed a test that supposedly could distinguish between sugar produced by flowering plants found in honey (called C3) and sugar made from either sugar-cane or corn/maize (called C4). The chemists thought they could pick up sugar adulteration in every sort honey using the test, but it now appears that the DHA/MGO conversion process naturally occurring in manuka honey creates a change in protein ratios that gives a false reading, once again proving that manuka honey is indeed a unique honey.*

In fact, the temperature the bees maintain in the hive was all-important. When the researchers held the honey at higher temperatures, both DHA and MGO levels actually went down, but the hydroxymethylfurfural levels (HMF, as you may recall) went up. And when HMF gets too high, it can no longer legally be defined as honey. We humans have 'over-cooked' it!

Sticky-fingers and counterfeits

The amazing discoveries of both MGO and DHA in manuka honey — substances that had previously eluded scientists for several decades, and which were then found by teams working on both sides of the world in the just a couple of years — showed several things.

First, fears that if the active ingredient in manuka honey was able to be identified, it would be a 'magic bullet' that pharmaceutical companies would be able to synthesise and patent, proved to be unfounded. Chemists already knew lots about MGO. What they didn't know, and had never realised, was that it could be part of a natural substance like manuka honey that allowed it to be a powerful antibiotic without being toxic. The real magic was how honey manages to do that. Secondly, there were now two means of being able to provide a standardised measurement of that activity. In fact, a company called Manuka Health was formed in New Zealand to market manuka honey using the MGO measurement system. It has provided support for the work Professor Henle and his team in Dresden continue to carry out on the subject.*

UMF™ and MGO are both valid methods of measuring the non-peroxide activity of manuka honey. One measures the activity itself, and the other measures the major compound producing that activity. Either, when the claim is subject to independent audit, should be enough to provide assurance to any consumer that they are getting what they pay for. Peter Molan has always said that a phenol equivalent activity of at least 10+ should be used in woundcare. Based on the correlation graph which Christopher Adams and the Waikato University team produced, that equates to about 263 milligrams per kilogram of MGO.*

The important thing is that people aren't fooled by other claims for 'activity', especially when it is being caused by hydrogen peroxide. That feature can be found in any honey, so no one should ever believe that it is 'unique'. The Unique Manuka Factor Honey Association, on the other hand, has done an excellent job in protecting its trademark, by ensuring that the appearance of the UMF brand on honey labels, as well as the phenol equivalence rating that is stated, are backed up internationally by independent testing and audits.

But what about manuka honey sold for other purposes, including honey from some of those manuka plant varieties which Jonathan Stephens found produced low levels of non-peroxide activity? An important aspect of manuka honey, which is sometimes overlooked in the rush to develop its therapeutic values, is its culinary aspects. Manuka honey has what the French call *cachet*, a term they use especially with their wine. It denotes a special group of prestigious qualities, including both sensory aspects and romance of place, or *terroir*. Manuka honey has something similar. It is often included as an ingredient in food products, and advertised on the label because of its ability to add value in a way that isn't often matched by other honeys. 'With clover honey added' somehow just doesn't have the same ring. For overseas consumers, the name also links directly to New Zealand, since the country is the only place in the world where significant amounts of the honey are produced.

The problem, though, is how to guarantee to the consumer that this honey is also 'wholly or mainly' manuka (to use the *Codex Alimentarius* term) even if it doesn't have a useful non-peroxide antibacterial rating? As we have seen, the traditional means of determining the floral source of manuka are not robust enough. Manuka isn't the only honey that is thixotropic; heather from the other side of the world is as well. Colour and flavour vary, and pollen content analysis can't differentiate between manuka and kanuka, two species that aren't in the same genus. Nevertheless, the stakes are high. Manuka honey is so expensive that security tags are put on jars to deter shop-lifters (who were described quite nicely in one newspaper article as 'sticky-fingered'). And a media outlet in the United Kingdom has even claimed that more manuka honey is being sold than New Zealand can produce.

There is no doubt that some honey is being labelled as manuka, either produced in New Zealand, or even overseas, that is knowingly counterfeit. Sadly this is to be expected, human nature (and the price of manuka honey) being what it is. At the same time, however, blending of floral sources does occur, not just during processing, but by the bees themselves. And this can be very hard to determine, even if you are a long-experienced beekeeper or a professional honey grader. Counterfeiting occurs in wine, too, but relying on the traditional means of honey analysis to tell you whether a honey is authentically manuka or not is like deciding what is a Bordeaux by gazing intently at its colour, swirling it around in your mouth, and spitting it into a silver pail. That sort of technique may appeal to *connoisseurs*, but the French now use sophisticated analytical machines to look for a wine type's particular chemical composition. And in the United States, scientists have even developed a simple sensor with colour-changing indicators that is able to distinguish between major wine varieties.*

Chemical analysis is surely the way manuka honey will soon be assessed for its authenticity as well, and scientists are using their skills and sensitive devices in an effort to find compounds that are unique to the honey — a chemical 'fingerprint'.

Honey and nectar — chicken and egg

Over 200,000 natural compounds have so far been found that can be used to determine one plant type from another. There are undoubtedly many more, especially since we have only looked seriously at about 1% of them, at least as far as their possible medicinal properties are concerned.

One of the major classifications of substances that might help us tell what flowering species honey bees have visited to produce their honey is the *phenolics*. Phenolics are a grouping that includes over 8000 natural compounds. One sub-set is the *flavonoids*, which have been much studied because of their many bioactive properties. They also happen to be important because they create at least some of the colours in both flower petals and pollen. Another sub-set of interest is the *phenolic acids*, a class of compounds manufactured by plants that are both essential for their growth, and also provide them with a strong defensive response against disease-causing pathogens. And a third is the *terpenes*, which give some plants their distinctive smell, and are the primary constituents of essential oils, including the ones that come from the manuka plant.

All three types of compound are associated with the immune systems of plants, and, while they are found in nectar, honey bees also collect them from trees and shrubs in the form of resin, combining them with beeswax, and using the result in their colonies as propolis. A recent chemical analysis identified seven such compounds for the first time in manuka honey.* Another phenolic compound called *methyl syringate* has also been found in manuka honey, and appears to be a powerful antioxidant. However, the compound has now been found in other, darker-coloured honeys as well.* A team lead by Jonathan Stephens has also looked at phenolic compounds in both manuka and kanuka honey, and found that, while they shared six phenolic acids, you could tell the honeys apart by the relative amounts of the acids they contained.*

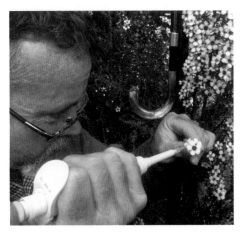

Researchers in both New Zealand and Japan have also found a marker substance that appears to be unique to *Leptospermum* honeys (manuka and jellybush). The compound has been tentatively named *leptosin*, and correlates with manuka honey's non-peroxide antibacterial activity.*

Another approach is to look at MGO itself. There is one record of MGO supposedly being found in kanuka honey, but the consensus now seems to be that MGO is confined to manuka and jellybush honey. Kanuka honey, on the other hand, has high levels of a compound called *methoxyphenyllactic acid.*

Dr Jonathan Stephens 'making like a bee' collecting manuka nectar with a pipette, the sort of painstaking work necessary to develop fingerprinting of honey types.

There is still a problem, though; a chicken-and-egg conundrum that we alluded to at the very beginning of this chapter. We can try to find substances to identify a particular honey, but how do we know for sure that the honey itself is totally from one plant species? Pure honey samples hardly ever occur. It is for this reason that researchers are also collecting nectar samples, and then comparing them to what is found in honey. In this case, DHA is a prime candidate, because in the work Christopher Adams carried out when he originally discovered that DHA in manuka honey changed into MGO, he didn't find any DHA in kanuka nectar.

Work is currently under way in New Zealand on just such a project. On behalf of The Unique Manuka Factor Honey Association, Jonathan Stephens and his team are 'making like honey bees' by painstakingly collecting thousands of nectar samples, as well as harvesting honey from hives that have been placed around the country in areas known to have dense stands of manuka. The project aims to 'accurately determine what manuka and other New Zealand mono-floral honeys actually are'.

A most extraordinary chain of events

When it comes to how we view honey, and therefore how we might go about analysing its source and makeup, manuka honey has changed the game. But much work still needs to be done. The science is one thing, but it may be even harder to convince those in positions of power and influence in the world that still hold fast to old notions of honey as nothing more than a food. Change in one sphere of human activity often doesn't transfer immediately to change elsewhere. In the case of manuka honey, however, it is essential that regulatory authorities come to grips with new methods of analysis, rather than falling back on the past.

We will never be able to replace honey bees in collecting nectar and transforming it into honey. But at least in mimicking the way they take it from flowers and then analysing the uniqueness of the compounds the nectar contains we may soon revolutionise how we are able to tell one honey from another. In the case of manuka honey, that may be as easy as measuring that one chemical called DHA which turns into another known as MGO.

Whatever the outcome, the story of manuka honey has been another truly amazing chapter in the relationship we have always had with honey bees, as well as the relationship both our species have with plants. And, as coincidences go, it would be hard to come up with a more remarkable set.

First, a special species of plant somehow managed to find its way from Australia to two big islands in the South Pacific, and once there liked the place so much that it grew in any number of different environments. Then many thousands of years later, brave groups of people in wind-borne canoes arrived on those islands, the last large landmass in the world settled by humans. And these people inadvertently helped that plant spread itself much more widely, clearing the way by burning large areas of the competing forest in the hunt for giant flightless birds.

Later, another group of people arrived, bringing with them an insect called the honey bee, an animal species that had never existed on those islands before. And the bees found that this special plant produced nectar very suitable for making a different sort of honey, the first honey ever produced in New Zealand. When that happened, a chemical in the nectar found itself in a new, acidic environment at just the right temperature, literally falling into the honey bees' 'cooking pot'. It was an environment it had never been in, and as a result it turned itself from one compound into another, a compound that had never appeared naturally in honey before.

Then eventually a scientist helped a friend test just one sample of that most peculiar honey, got a result that didn't seem right, and because he was so inquisitive he looked at a lot more samples as well. He found a new antibacterial activity in that honey, told the public about it, and then perhaps even more importantly realised just how powerful it could be in human health. As a result, the honey broke new ground for a natural product, becoming a woundcare dressing accepted by mainstream medicine.

Finally, almost three decades later, the 'magic ingredient' and its very close relation were found. By then manuka, a honey once very neglected, was truly famous around the world.

It was a long chain of events so extraordinary it almost seems miraculous. And no one would ever look at honey, one of the amazing gifts that honey bees offer us, in quite the same way again.

Epilogue

DISAPPEARING BEES, THE PRICE OF HONEY AND MAINTAINING A SACRED FLAME

The idea that honey bees are disappearing from the planet has become one of the great memes of the new millennium. No matter where you live in the world you have probably heard about the problem, and maybe even worry about it at least a bit. A meme, on the other hand, might not be a term you've ever come across before. The evolutionary biologist Richard Dawkins first came up with the idea of memes back in the 1970s in his book *The Selfish Gene*. A *meme* is a new word, gesture or idea that is to cultural change what a mutation might be to evolution. And like mutations, we somehow collectively and almost sub-consciously select ones that appear to be useful, while eventually discarding those that don't.

Memes can be really big ideas, or very small turns of phrase. Examples of memes include adoption of the abbreviation 'OK' by almost every culture and language around the world, the idea that freedom is a universal human right, and even simple proverbs like 'the early bird catches the worm'. A meme works a bit like gossip, at least at the beginning. It starts out being shared between a couple of people, but pretty soon we all start talking about it. Eventually it just becomes part of what everybody knows. Memes only happen with some special pieces of information, while the rest just seem to come and quickly go in the steady stream of what we see and hear each day. What makes it a meme is when one of those ideas 'clicks' and literally 'goes global'. We may not be able to say where we first heard it or when, but a meme ends up firmly fixed in the minds of people in every corner of the world. There is nothing derogatory about the term. Memes may be true or false, or even neither. Only time can tell for sure. But what is fascinating is how they enter and often alter our culture. They are a remarkable social phenomenon, one that has become far more rapid and prolific now that the world is connected by instant communication and the internet.

The origins of the disappearing honey bees meme can be traced to a problem beekeepers in the United States first identified in their hives in the winter of 2006–2007. Honey bee colonies sometimes die over winter, often due to starvation. Try as they might, beekeepers occasionally misjudge how much honey needs to be left on a hive. As for wild colonies, unless a swarm manages to find a nest site big enough to allow for the storage of ample honey reserves, death over winter or in early spring is often the norm.

That particular winter, however, something was different. Much larger numbers of bee colonies were dying, and in some cases there was still honey left in the combs. The worker bees just seemed to have disappeared, leaving behind a small group of bees attending to the queen. Scientists called in to study the problem couldn't come up with a definitive cause. The term 'colony collapse disorder' was coined to describe it; 'disorder' because no particular disease could be confirmed.

Varroa, the dreaded parasitic mite that was devastating honey bee colonies around the world, seemed to be part of the problem, but the symptoms weren't quite what beekeepers normally associated with the pest. Viruses were also implicated, because varroa is in many ways a crawling hypodermic syringe, sucking the blood of honey bees, and in the process injecting viruses, some of which had never been a significant problem with honey bees before.

Beekeepers, particularly in Europe, blamed another culprit, a new group of insecticides called *neonicotinoids* that are both long-lasting in the plants that have been treated with them, and also interfere with the navigational systems of insects that feed on those plants, including honey bees that collect the plants' nectar and pollen.

Reports of large losses of honey bee colonies began to appear in the press, and before long the story started to take on epic proportions. Each year it seemed that 30%, 40% or even 50% of beehives were dying over winter. And people everywhere began to wake up to the fact that bees did more than just make honey.

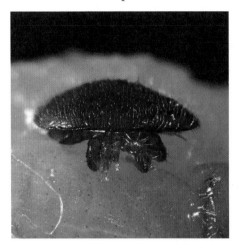

Varroa destructor (the 'vampire' mite), the reason honey bees in most places now must depend on humans for their survival.

A realisation dawned that honey bees were far more important because of the pollination they carried out, and concerns began to be expressed about threats to the world's food supply.

Then someone found a supposed quote from Albert Einstein, arguably the most brilliant person who ever lived, saying that if honey bees disappeared off the face of the earth humans would only have four years left to live. As a result, around the globe people began to fear we were facing a bee-related Armageddon. Honey bees, and their significance to mankind, had come to the forefront of human consciousness. A new meme was well and truly planted in all our brains.

Investigating the disappearing bees meme

Our rags-to-riches biography of manuka honey is now more or less complete. But before we finish it is perhaps worth taking a few pages to look at this disappearing bees meme a bit more closely, especially now that we have learned more about honey bees and that special relationship our two species share.

Knowledge is strength, especially when it comes to confronting an issue that is both highly emotional and seemingly unsolvable. And there are perhaps some insights to be gained about the future of both honey bees and beekeeping from what has happened to manuka honey in New Zealand over the past several decades. In fact, we may even be able to see a way forward, one that requires more than anything a change in our behaviour as consumers, rather than simply just wringing our hands in despair.

The first thing we need to do is put the role of honey bees and our food supply in its proper perspective. While insect pollination is crucial, both to thousands of flowering plant species, and to a much smaller number that produce some of the foods we eat, the plants that contribute to the bulk of our diet don't fall into that category. These are the staples like wheat, rice, corn/maize, and the coarse grains such as oats, barley, etc. They make up two-thirds of the volume of crops we grow around the world each year, either as food to eat directly, or as feed for the animals that we then go on to eat. These are the very select number of plant species that humanity truly cannot do without. But in each case they are pollinated entirely by the wind. Bees don't play a direct role in putting bread on the table or rice in a bowl, nor are they essential for the beef in the middle of a hamburger bun, or the pork that adds flavour and protein to a stir fry.

Bees instead make it possible for us to have a bountiful cornucopia of other foods. They do this indirectly in many instances by helping to create the seeds planted to grow a range of vegetables we put on our plates (although a number of important crops like potatoes aren't part of that list). And insect pollination is also responsible for a variety of the fruits we have for dessert (but not many of the tropical varieties like bananas, or wind-pollinated ones like grapes). There are even some crops, like strawberries and coffee for example, that while not absolutely needing insect pollination for fruit set, nevertheless have improved yields when their flowers are visited by bees.

So to put it in its most basic form, without honey bees life would be a lot less tasty, but despite what Einstein may (or may not) have said, we wouldn't starve to death. In fact, a recent study suggests that with the loss of *all* pollinators (not just honey bees), agricultural production around the world would decrease by about 8%.*

This is not to say, however, that the problem of disappearing bees isn't still serious, especially for many people in the more industrialised, higher-income parts of the world who take that cornucopia spilling out onto their tables as a matter of right. In fact, it is in the places where we have become the most efficient at producing large amounts of the highest-quality fruits and vegetables that we have become most reliant on honey bees, and also where currently those bees seem to be most at risk.

We have fine-tuned our palates, and committed our vast horticultural production resources to a narrow range of fruits and vegetables, many of which evolved in the same temperate regions of the world where honey bees also first originated. The bees long ago developed an intense, mutually beneficial relationship with those plants. And we humans are now part of a co-evolutionary *ménage à trois*.

Commercial pollination and industrialised horticulture — hand in hand

Honey bees have become crucial in the commercial production of pip-fruit like apples, stone-fruit like peaches, and, most famously, nuts like almonds. Early each spring in California, over 60% of the beehives in the United States are trucked into almond orchards. The hives then make their way to other crops in a commercial pollination industry that sometimes sees colonies of honey bees transported in a number of stages many thousands of miles around the country each year.

But what most people don't realise is how recent the development of commercial pollination is. For many centuries when we weren't so 'efficient' in this sort of food production, horticulture was part of a more diverse sort of agriculture. It was, in fact, still part of a 'natural' ecosystem of sorts. We certainly made major alterations to it, slimming down the number of species, improving plants we found useful and tasty, and weeding out those we did not. But we weren't overly concerned with spots on our fruit, or even if we could have it fresh whenever we wanted it, no matter what time of the year. And crucially, we grew most things on small, mixed farms, with uncultivated and often wild places where pollinating insects could live right nearby.

All that changed with the advent of scientific horticulture, particularly after World War II. We wanted to produce more and better. We did it with mechanisation, routine spraying of agricultural chemicals, and huge acreages of not just one species, but often a single, cloned variety of plant. We made growing things 'industrial', and we wanted to be able to control every input we could. But when we did so, it eventually became evident that some of those fruits and vegetables still needed an important part of the old ecosystem. Insects were required to pollinate the flowers, set the seed and trigger production of the crop. Growers used to rely on the apiary down the road, or the wild pollinating insects that lived in the weeds, hedgerows or nearby wood lot. But now the weeds had been sprayed out, the hedgerows pulled up, and the wood lot chopped down to make way for greater acreages of the valuable crops. There were hardly any nest sites left for those insects, and any that still managed to find a home were likely to be killed by the sprays used to keep the crops free from pests.

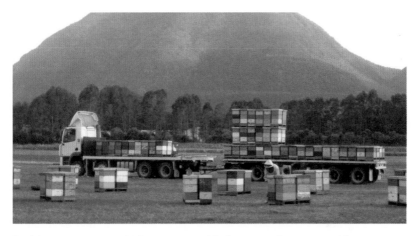

Beehives are now routinely transported in large numbers to provide pollination for the vast acreages of monoculture that make up today's industrialised horticulture.

The beekeeper, meantime, had moved his apiary away. There were no longer enough species of plants around, flowering in sequence over enough months of the season, for the honey bee colonies to properly sustain themselves, let alone bring in the surplus honey the beekeeper needed to make a living. And the insecticides were just too dangerous. The orchard may have been down the road on another property, but you can never control where honey bees will fly. So commercial pollination, the insertion of populous colonies of suitable insects that are easy to control and transport, began in earnest in the late 1960s, just as industrialised horticulture began to take over, particularly in North America. And for beekeepers who became involved, it meant major change. Now they kept their hives away from the big plantations, and brought them in just as the flowers begin to bloom, taking the hives back out again a few weeks later.

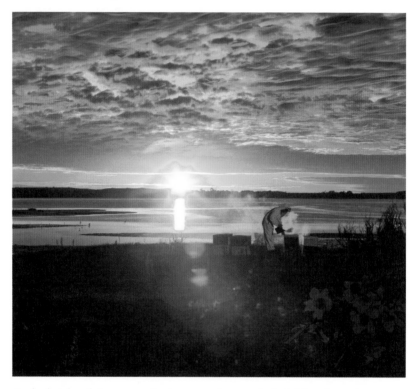

At the height of the season, beekeepers often work their hives from dawn to dusk, and also move them into orchards at night, once the bees have all returned to the hive.

Beekeeping is a tough business, full of hot, hard work. But pollination made it just that much tougher. Beekeepers found themselves working late into the night, because if you moved your beehives during the day you left many of the foraging bees behind. And much more co-ordination was required, not just into and out of orchards, but also onto the next crop, as well as maintaining places to keep the hives once the pollination season was over.* In such circumstances, it was inevitable that beekeepers would start charging a substantial price for pollination services. The stress on both the beekeepers and the bees became significant, especially when the colonies were shifted from one monoculture to another, and were often shut up for long periods as they rode on massive trailers pulled by semi-trucks, sometimes for days at a time. Finally, when you added something as troubling as colony collapse disorder to the equation, a problem that the scientists couldn't seem to solve, the question eventually became: will there be enough hives in areas with industrialised horticulture to meet demand?

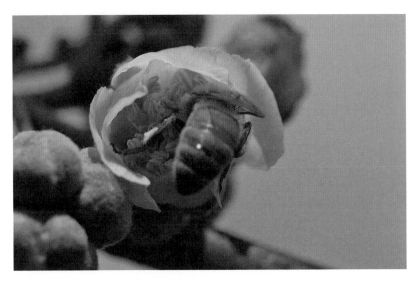

A honey bee gathering pollen from a just-opening kiwifruit flower.

It is important to understand that the scope of the pollination problem isn't the same everywhere you go. It is confined to the parts of the world where the mostly temperate crops requiring honey bee pollination can be grown, and then only where the systems of production have become big, controlled and monocultural. This is certainly the case in many parts of the United States, and especially in California, where over a third of the nation's vegetables and two-thirds of its fruits and nuts are produced.* In those places the pollination 'system' would seem to have now become very fragile indeed. But even in a country like New Zealand, commercial pollination has become a crucial necessity for the many hectares of kiwifruit that are grown cheek-by-jowl.

The mite that needs the bee that needs us

The effect of varroa on honey bees, on the other hand, is far more universal. As we have seen, over the past 300 years people have spread honey bees from their natural domiciles in Europe and Africa to every continent except Antarctica. And the bees' drastic increase in numbers has owed much to the beekeepers who were determined to make their living from their hives.

No one knows how many honey bee colonies there might have been before we started keeping them. But it is obvious that those numbers would have fluctuated widely in various areas as a result of extremes in weather conditions, including longer and harsher winters than normal, and, even more crucially, terribly inclement springs. And it would have taken a number of good foraging years before one or two swarms issuing from a colony annually would have returned population numbers to previous levels. The chances of survival for honey bee colonies would have improved at least somewhat when we started keeping them in clay pots and skeps, but we couldn't assess their condition very accurately, replace their queens when needed, or properly treat them for disease.

That all changed with those moveable frame hives. Once they came along in the middle of the nineteenth century, beekeeping grew remarkably around the world, and with it there occurred a significant increase in *Apis mellifera* as a species. This certainly continued to be the case right through the period of the development of industrialised agriculture, especially as we altered our landscapes and took away many of the natural nesting sites that honey bees would have needed to maintain colonies on their own. There were still wild colonies, but the large number of honey bees in the environment in the more developed parts of the world owed much to beekeepers who were not just looking after honey bees so well, but giving them many more suitable places to live in than they would be able to find in nature.

With the advent of varroa, however, the mutually beneficial relationship we have always had with honey bees has become something entirely more crucial. In effect, the mite took advantage of the human–bee relationship, and has moved on the backs of honey bees, most often transported by beekeepers themselves, from the mite's original habitat to every major beekeeping country in the world except Australia, in the process hugely extending its range and population as well.*

Varroa may originally have been a parasite of *Apis cerana,* another honey bee species confined to eastern Asia, but ironically it has now become completely dependent in all those new locales not just on *Apis mellifera*, but also on the people who keep them. Parasites never kill their host, but varroa and *Apis mellifera* don't have that sort of relationship. The mite can't help but kill that species of honey bee, so for it to continue to exist in those places it needs beekeepers to keep making up the colony losses it creates.

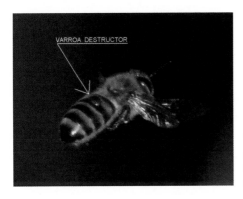

Varroa can easily hitch a ride on worker bees, giving the mite a remarkable ability to infest new hives.

As a result, all three creatures (bees, varroa and humans) are now locked in a dangerous sort of dance. We want and need honey bees, and varroa can't help but like them, too. As for *Apis mellifera*, they absolutely can no longer do without their human friends. We are no longer just their benefactor. At this moment in time, without the treatments we give honey bee colonies to control populations of varroa, all those colonies will surely die.

No one knows how long it will take before honey bees develop a level of resistance to that parasite sufficient enough to allow them to exist as wild creatures once again. It has been less than a century since honey bees first came into contact with the pest. And natural selection in an organism that procreates not truly as individual bees, but through the production of 'super-organisms' called colonies, just doesn't work that fast.

As for 'artificial' selection (the term Darwin once used to describe human-assisted changes in plants and animals), unfortunately it isn't as easy to breed honey bees to take on desirable new traits as it is with cows or sheep. In nature, honey bee queens and drones mate high in the air. You can control their mating through the use of instrumental insemination, but the technique is painstaking, and as a result it is not economically viable to produce the many thousands needed by commercial beekeepers. And of course when a colony headed by an instrumentally inseminated queen decides to produce a replacement, as is always their natural inclination to do, the new virgin queen will mate in an uncontrolled manner high in the air again. Honey bees insist on living by the motto 'don't fence me in', and under current circumstances that is a real barrier to overcoming the varroa problem once and for all. As a result, for the foreseeable future it will be up to humans to look after their honey bee partners. Without us, it is quite possible that they might not survive.

Disappearing bees or disappearing beekeepers?

What you have heard so far must seem hopeless, and no doubt that is one of the reasons so many media articles on the subject concentrate on the doom and gloom. But rest assured, all is not lost. Far from it in fact. And here is where we can perhaps learn something from what happened with manuka honey in New Zealand. While many of those stories report on the continuing losses of beehives in the United States and Europe of over 30% per year, few mention a very important fact that should be obvious to anyone who even thinks for a moment about the maths: beekeepers, and especially those who rely on bees to make a living, are experts at replacing those losses, growing out new colonies by splitting existing ones. With the right conditions and good management, professional beekeepers are often able to double their number of live hives in a six-week period in the spring.

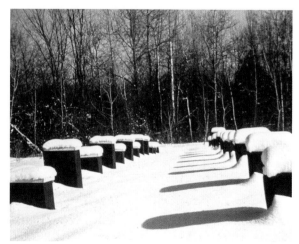

With human help, honey bees have spread all around the globe, and can even survive in cold climates where it would be almost impossible for large numbers of colonies to exist on their own from one year to the next.

Analysis of hive census data from around the world, as incomplete and possibly inaccurate as it is, also suggests that global hive stocks have increased by over 60% since varroa began to spread in the early 1960s. World honey production also seems to have increased, by about 8%, since the first reports of colony collapse disorder. So what's going on?* The big problem is that, while there are more hives in the world than perhaps ever before, hive numbers in some regions, and particularly in the more industrialised areas like the United States and some parts of Europe, have gone down. And as it turns out, the problem in those places isn't just disappearing bees, it's disappearing beekeepers.

In many less developed parts of the world, beekeeping is seen as a worthwhile way to make a living (provided of course you can take the stings!). You don't need much capital, you don't have to own land, and you can increase your colonies once you learn the right techniques. As the amazing success of beekeeping development in the past 50 years has shown, especially in countries like China and Argentina, compared with many of the alternatives, being a commercial beekeeper isn't all that bad.

In a place like the United States, however, where the biggest need exists for commercial pollination, but where sufficient hive numbers to do the job are most at risk, the situation is much different. There are lots of well-paid alternative forms of employment, especially ones where you don't have to work as hard or as long. The problem is compounded by the fact that major food manufacturers and supermarket chains often decide not to buy bulk commodity honey from the country's beekeepers simply because it is marginally more expensive.

The economy is something of an ecosystem, too, and if US beekeepers struggle to make a go of it because they can't achieve a reasonable profit from the honey they have to extract and process, they are less likely to want to carry on, regardless of how important their bees are for the pollination of the nation's crops. You don't spend hours removing heavy boxes of honey from your hives, and even more hours in the shed removing it from the combs, just to 'break even'. Those beekeepers are faced with higher costs, lower relative returns, and the inability to attract good labour. There is a huge disconnect between their lifestyle and what they see all around them. The end result is that there just isn't a very strong incentive to grow out new hives and replace dead ones. On the contrary, when it comes time for commercial beekeepers to retire, their children aren't usually interested in taking over, and it can even be hard to get someone to buy their hives.

In New Zealand, on the other hand, a country with a developed economy and an enviable standard of living, something very different has happened. Beekeepers in that country experienced varroa for the first time in 2000, and there was an adjustment for a time as they learned how to control the pest. The mite eventually killed all the wild colonies in the North Island, in the process virtually eliminating the European black bee variety that made up the bulk of those feral stocks, the very descendants of the sort of honey bees that Mary Bumby first brought to Mangungu over a century and a half earlier. But since that time, while the media has reported hive numbers going down in the United States and parts of Europe, New Zealand beekeepers have increased their hive numbers from 290,000 in 2005 to over 450,000 in 2013. At the same time, a honey that beekeepers in the country previously had a hard time selling is now worth $140 million per year. It hardly needs to be stated, but obviously those hive increases and the price of manuka honey are intimately linked.

In a world that for good reason feels saddened and sometimes even fearful about the future of this special relationship we humans have always had with honey bees, especially now that our industrial food-growing systems have made us more dependent than ever on the pollination services provided by hives managed by commercial beekeepers, what has happened with the dramatic increase in hive numbers in New Zealand shows there is a way forward. Bees don't need to disappear, even though they can no longer survive in many parts of the world without care from those commercial beekeepers. If we are prepared to pay the prices for bee products that these beekeepers need to make a good living, our story shows that the numbers of honey bee colonies can actually increase, rather than inevitably go down.

The story of manuka honey in New Zealand is, above all else, a story of hope for the future. But we have to put our money where our concern is, rather than simply pay lip service to it. The big question, though, is what can the average person do? Many people have now become so interested in honey bees that they are contemplating buying their own hives. There are plenty of excellent reasons to keep a hive or two, including learning about these fascinating creatures, providing pollination for your home gardens and those of your nearby neighbours, and of course making a bit of honey for yourself.

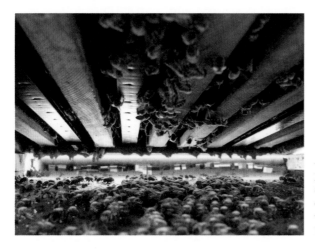

A remarkable picture that gives a 'bees-eye' view of the outside world from the bottom of a hive.

But don't kid yourself, or those around you. The problem of disappearing bees, at least as it relates to industrialised food production, isn't going to be solved by hobbyists putting a few beehives in their backyards, no matter how many and how well-intentioned they are. It would take a village of people keeping one or two hives each to match the number of hives kept by one average-sized commercial beekeeper. And with our modern systems of horticulture, and those vast acreages of single crops like apples or almonds, it is only the people with large numbers of hives and the wherewithal to transport them that can really get the job done. But for that to happen, particularly in parts of the world that are more highly developed and have higher incomes, commercial beekeeping must be seen in the future as an option comparable with other skilled activities. Being a commercial beekeeper requires dedication and a forgoing of many of modern life's benefits. It is a sacrifice that, if we are honest with ourselves, most of us are not prepared to make. So now, more than ever before, we have to give these people their due. Having a couple of beehives in the backyard can be a satisfying pastime. But what the world needs now and into the future are large numbers of well-kept hives that only people dedicating their lives to the venture can hope to provide.

It's payback time

Humans have always had an important relationship with honey bees, but in the past several hundred years we have greatly increased their number as we have developed and changed the globe. These amazing insects have given us honey, and other bee products, and pollinated the crops we have brought with us from many parts of the world, allowing us to greatly vary our diet and produce more fruits and vegetables more cheaply by growing them in an industrialised, monocultural way.

But now we must pay the bees back, because without them remaining in abundance, especially in many of the places where they were never present originally, this modern agricultural system we have created can't carry on. The relationship we humans have had with bees for so long has become one of mutual need, exacting in a way that it has never been since the time, at the dawn of our species, when we, as nomadic hunter-gathers, first came upon them. Honey bees have become necessary to us, and we are absolutely essential to them. We are now inextricably linked.

Because of varroa, honey bees can no longer exist as wild creatures in most parts of the world. As a result, beekeepers (and particularly commercial beekeepers, because they are responsible for the vast bulk of honey bee colonies) have become the modern equivalent of an ancient priesthood, whose job it once was to maintain a flame forever burning in the temple. Now, however, that flame is the honey bee, and the temple is the food-giving environment we all live in.

It may make us feel better about ourselves to occasionally take a minute in our cluttered lives to worry about the disappearing bees. And we can even go so far as to stop and give thanks to honey bees and their commercial keepers the next time we pull out an apple and take that delicious first bite. But in the end, doing something about it requires at least casting an economic vote. Beekeepers around the world don't necessarily need more manuka honeys. But what they do require, and in long run what all us who depend on bees to pollinate the foods we like to eat need as well, is for everyone to buy more of all of the honeys that are produced around the world, and at higher prices.

For much of our human history, honey has been a major source of sweetness in our diet, and an important provider of medicine as well. All that has changed in the modern world. Today the total world production of honey represents less than 1% of all the sugar we consume each year. But in the future, it doesn't have to continue to be that way. In fact, if everyone in the world ate a tablespoon of honey each day, we would consume the entire world's annual honey production in less than three weeks.*

So buy more honey, and use it a lot more. Seek out recipes that call for honey, put it in your coffee and tea, make your very own energy drinks. But don't just look for the cheapest price. Check out the label, see where it comes from, who produced it, what floral sources it contains. And go on, buy an expensive one. Think of it as your offering to those modern-day versions of the ancient priests — the beekeepers keeping alive the spirit of our age-old relationship with honey bees.

NOTES

Chapter 1: THE SAMPLE THAT DIDN'T MAKE SENSE

Page 16: '... circular glass dishes developed by his friend Julius Petri.' For more information about Robert Koch and Julius Petri, see Koch's biography at *Nobelprize.org*.

Page 16: '... and in so doing coined the term "magic bullet" '. For more information about Paul Ehrlich, see his biography at *Nobelprize.org*.

Page 17: For more information on the development of bacterial testing methods see Poupard, J. et al. (1994).

Page 17: '... we are only a small part of theirs', and the paragraphs that follow. See Bryson, B. (2003), Chapter 20, 'Small World'.

Page 18: '... we have had telephones and lights in our homes ...'. See Bryson, B. (2010), pages 370, 394.

Page 19: 'Kerry Simpson didn't think anything more about his little experiment.' Peter Molan has always acknowledged the role Kerry Simpson played in the discovery of the special non-peroxide antibacterial activity of manuka honey. See, for instance, Molan, P. (2012a). In an interview with the author in November, 2013, Peter said, 'If I ever get around to writing my book on manuka honey, I'll make sure to dedicate it to Kerry.'

Page 21: For information on the introduction of thyme to New Zealand, see Wilkinson, E. et al. (1979).

Page 21: For information on the introduction of heather to New Zealand, see Bagnall, A. (1982).

Page 24: '*S. aureus* proved to be a perfect organism in this regard ...'. See Molan, P. and Russell, K. (1988).

Page 26: '... testing for her Master's of Science thesis.' See Russell, K. (1983).

Page 26: 'The first, by Peter, Mary Smith and Murray Reid ...'. See Molan, P. et al. (1988).

Page 26: 'The second, written by Peter and Kate Russell ...'. See Molan, P. and Russell, K. (1988).

Page 26: 'Finally in 1991 another paper was published, this time in a well-known international journal ...'. See Allen, K. et al. (1991).

Chapter 2: YOU NEVER CAN TELL WITH BEES

Page 31: For more information on ancient records of honey hunting and beekeeping, see Crane, E. (1983).

Page 32: '... represented the harvest from probably at least 5000 clay hives.' See Crane, E. (1975), page 456.

Page 32: 'The author Michael Pollan has argued that maize "used" humans ...'. See Pollan, M. (2006), Chapter 1, 'The Plant: Corn's Conquest'.

Page 34: There are many books on the subject of the social behaviour of bees, but the classic is Michner, C. (1974). Try also Seeley, T. (2009).

Page 35: '... when scientists used harmonic radar to track bees ...'. See Riley, J. et al. (2005).

Page 37: The idea of business learning from ecosystems, and the concept of 'up-cycling', is described in McDonough, W. and Braungart, M. (2002).

Page 37: '... it's a set of processes we often lump together under the general term "cooking".' For a wonderful discourse on the idea of human transformation of food, see Pollan, M. (2013).

Page 42: One of the classic reviews of what goes on in a honey bee colony is Winston, M. (1987). For a more recent survey, try Caron, D. et al. (2013).

Page 45: '... proved for the first time that honey bees really do use propolis to self-medicate'. See Simone-Finstrom, M. and Spivak, M. (2012).

Page 46: '... crucial element in the move from a hunter-gatherer nomadic lifestyle to a more sedentary existence.' See Lévi-Strauss, C. (1974).

Page 49: Uses of honey in ancient civilisations: there are a number of good reviews on the subject, including especially Crane, E. (1999).

Page 50: 'The medicinal uses of bee products are described in the Divine Farmer's Materia Medica (Shennong Bencao Jing).' See Yang, S. (1998).

Page 51: 'Aboriginal tribes consider honey to be the supreme delicacy ...'. See Low, T. (1989).

Page 51: 'As Eva Crane, the world's foremost authority on honey, has said ...'. Crane, E. (1975), page 465.

Page 51: '... a recent re-evaluation of the evidence suggests that may not have been the case.' In fact, evidence from the Stone Age, Antiquity, the Middle Ages and early Modern times suggests that ordinary people ate much larger quantities of honey than has previously been acknowledged. See Allsop, K. and Miller, J. (1996).

Page 52: '... in the German city of Meissen mead (or at least honey beer) was used to put out a fire ...'. See Crane, E. (1980), page 94.

Page 52: '... sugary substance in northern Europe' (used in the brewing of beer). See Hornsey, I. (2003).

Page 52: '... advent of the moveable frame hive, popularised (if not perhaps actually invented) by the Reverend L. L. Langstroth ...'. Langstroth promoted the moveable frame hive, and 'bee space' (the gap of ⅜ inch/9.5 millimetre between combs that bees will not fill with beeswax) that made it all work, in The Hive and The Honey Bee, first published in 1853. The book has been updated and reprinted many times since, and the 1992 edition (Graham, 1992) is arguably the most comprehensive book on the science and craft of beekeeping that has so far been produced. The 'Eureka!' quote from Langstroth's diary appears in that book.

Page 54: 'For instance, in New Zealand it was part of standard woundcare practice in hospitals prior to World War II.' Interview with Peter Molan, November 2013.

Page 54: '... honey itself was shown to be antibacterial as far back as 1892 ...'. The discovery was made by the Dutch scientist van Ketel (van Ketel, B., 1892).

Page 54: '... in 1969 the US Surgeon General could confidently state, "The time has come to close the book on infectious disease." ' See Nelson, R. (2003).

Page 54: '... sugar production worldwide had now displaced honey by a factor of 100 to 1 ...'. In 2011–12, world honey production was 1.6 million tonnes, while sugar production was 168 million tonnes. Source: *FAOStat*.

Page 55: '... They have been around a lot longer than we have (several billion years longer, in fact) ...'. See Wacey, D. et al. (2011).

Chapter 3: GIVING THE STUFF AWAY

Page 57: The story of beekeeping on Great Barrier Island is told in two documents. The first is an entertaining pamphlet, *A History of Honey Production on Great Barrier Island,* produced by Dave Watson of The Milk, Honey and Grain Museum, Claris, Great Barrier Island. The second is 'Les & Beverley's Story', published in the magazine *New Zealand Memories* (June/July 2008). Les Blackwell also very kindly shared his memories of beekeeping on Great Barrier Island in an interview with the author in December 2013.

Page 58: 'While even today manuka (and its close relative kanuka) make up almost half of the vegetation on the island ...'. See Great Barrier Island Charitable Trust (2010).

Page 58: 'Even as early as 1910 it was fetching a market price of 4 pence a pound, while "bush" sold for half that amount.' See 'On The Land' (1910).

Page 60: '... in what the English naturalist David Bellamy calls "Moa's Ark"...'. See Bellamy, D. et al. (1990). As we will see in a subsequent chapter, however, not all the plants and animals we take for granted as being passengers on that 'ark' have been along for the journey the whole time.

Page 60: The mission house at Mangungu is maintained by the New Zealand Historic Places Trust. After it played its role in the founding of the country, and the introduction of honey bees, however, the two-storey building travelled around a bit. In 1855 it was taken to pieces and moved (by sea) to the Auckland suburb of Onehunga, where it was first a Methodist parsonage, and then sold to private owners in 1921. In 1972 it was dismantled once again, trucked in sections back up to the Hokianga, and both faithfully and beautifully restored by the Trust. Many of the stories about Mary Bumby and her brother John (and great pictures of how the house made its way back home) are included in documents on display in the house.

Page 63: The best compilation of accounts of Mary Bumby's introduction of honey bees to New Zealand is in an article that appeared in *The New Zealand Beekeeper* (Dawson, C. 1979). Mary and James Bumby embarked on the *James* at Gravesend on 16 August 1838, and reached Hokianga on 18 March 1839, with a stop of 36 days at Hobart, where the bees no doubt had time to recuperate and feed on the local flowering plants, since it was the height of summer.

Page 64: By far the most thorough and well-documented account of how honey bees were introduced into both New Zealand and Australia, as well as descriptions of what beekeeping was like in those early days, can be found in Barrett, P. (1995). According to Barrett, honey bees were first established in Australia when hives from England were landed at Port Jackson (the bay that contains Sydney harbour) on 9 March 1822.

Page 64: 'They have increased to such an extent, as to have become wild and fill the forest ...'. See Taylor, R. (1868).

Page 64: The Reverend William Charles Cotton's first book on beekeeping, *My Bee Book*, was written in 1839, before he left for New Zealand, and was published in 1842. Following his arrival, he also published *A Manual for New Zealand Beekeepers*, in 1848. Both books provide details on transporting honey bee colonies by ship. See Barrett, P. (1995).

Page 65: 'Before the introduction of the honey bee they had to send over to England every year for white clover seed ...'. *British Beekeeping Journal*, as quoted in Hopkins, I. (1886).

Page 65: '... offered one of the hives upon safe completion of the trip.' *The New Zealand Journal* (1842). As reported in Barrett, P. (1995).

Page 66: '... dock in Honolulu at daybreak, and not leave again before nightfall ...'. Mackay, A. (1893) *The Australian Bee Bulletin*. As reported in Barrett, P. (1995).

Page 66: A concise history of beekeeping in New Zealand can be found in the pages of *Practical Beekeeping in New Zealand*, 4th edition (2011), written by Andrew Matheson and Murray Reid, and published by Exisle.

Page 67: Books by Isaac Hopkins included *The New Zealand Bee Manual* (1881), *The Australasian Bee Manual* (1882; 1925), *The Illustrated Australasian Bee Manual and Complete Guide to Modern Bee Culture in the Southern Hemisphere* (1886; 1904), and *Forty-two Years of Beekeeping in New Zealand* (1916).

Page 69: Details about American foulbrood and its control in New Zealand are the subject of *Control of American Foulbrood Without the Use of Drugs*. The first edition of this book (Goodwin and Van Eaton, 1999) was published by the National Beekeepers' Association of New Zealand. Along with being an expert in American foulbrood and the varroa mite, Mark Goodwin is also one of the world's leading pollination scientists.

Page 70: The story of Robert Gibbs and 'Beeswing', the house built on one year's honey crop, is told in a delightful pamphlet of beekeeping reminiscences, *Bees in Their Bonnets*, by Lennon, W. (1948).

Page 74: '... it was becoming evident that in future manuka honey would be very difficult to sell ...'. See Anonymous (1951).

Page 74: 'Manuka honey cannot be clarified or blended with other honey by the usual methods.' See Anonymous (1953).

Page 74: '... in the hopes that 'the resulting product (invert sugar) will find a demand for manufacturing purposes.' See Horticulture Division (1951).

Page 76: '... warned against the establishment of apiaries close to manuka areas ...'. Winter, T. (1962).

Page 76: Details about the thixotropic characteristics of manuka and heather honey can be found in Eva Crane's famous work, *Honey: A Comprehensive Survey* (Crane, E., 1975).

Page 79: For more details on the package bee trade from New Zealand to Canada, see www.packagebees.co.nz/how.htm.

Page 79: Malcolm Haines's prophetic comments made at the Taupo conference on honey marketing can be found in Haines, M. (1975).

Page 80: 'It argued quite forcefully in an information circular to beekeeper suppliers that, while the export market for retail packs could not be ignored ...'. See Honey Marketing Authority (1967).

Page 81: For a fascinating look into the disputes that raged within the New Zealand beekeeping industry regarding the HMA, it is worthwhile reading the reports and remits to NBA conferences, beginning in 1976, as reported in *The New Zealand Beekeeper* magazine. The HMA came to a halt in 1982.

Page 81: In the United States, the Food, Conservation, and Energy Act (2008) authorises non-recourse marketing assistance loans (MALs) and loan deficiency payments (LDPs) through the Commodity Credit Corporation.

Page 81: Legislation creating the EC apiculture support programmes are contained in articles 105–110 of Council Regulation (EC) No. 1234/2007. The programmes are obviously subject to both review and change, and not all member states make payments directly to beekeepers, most notably the United Kingdom.

Page 82: 'Some might argue that what happened with honey in New Zealand was a free market revolution ...'. Deregulation of honey exports was even used as a test case by agricultural economists in the country when they were investigating whether other producer boards should be abolished (although as we shall see, results in the beekeeping industry were decidedly mixed in the early years). See, for instance, Ward, A. (1986).

Chapter 4: THE PRESS RELEASE THAT GREW LEGS

Page 83: Actual copies of the original manuka honey press release that grew legs and travelled around the world are pretty hard to come by, since it was produced before the digital era. It does appear to have been more or less recorded in its entirety, however, in the pages of *Buzzwords*, a newsletter once produced for the National Beekeepers' Association of New Zealand. The release was issued on 22 November 1991, while the *Buzzwords* article was published in February 1992.

Page 84: The story about Peter Molan being interviewed by *Cosmopolitan* magazine comes from an interview he had with the author in November 2013.

Page 87: There are a number of publications having to do with the National Beekeepers' Association's Pest Management Strategy for American foulbrood, mostly held in the archives of the association. The author was the primary consultant hired by the association to help with its development. A number of association members gave freely of their time and energy in the process. Their steadfastness, and the support of an overwhelming percentage of association members, is no doubt the primary reason the strategy was eventually approved.

Page 88: The industry plans of the beekeepers' association from 1980s and early 1990s are also contained in various issues of *The New Zealand Beekeeper*, and in the association archives.

Page 90: Bill Floyd's address to the association conference in 1991 was published in *The New Zealand Beekeeper* in spring of that year (Floyd, B., 1991).

Page 92: A good description of mountain beech and its honeydew-producing scale can be found in Morales, G. et al. (1988).

Page 92: *New Zealand Honey Sensory Profiles — Monofloral Varieties*, was published by the New Zealand Honey Food and Ingredient Advisory Service in February 1997.

Page 94: The amazing life story of the founder of Comvita is recorded in *100 Years of Claude Stratford* (Avery, B., 2010). It is a testament to the old adage, 'If at once you don't succeed, try, try and try again!' Comvita's website is www.comvita.com

Page 95: The Reg Day story appeared on the TV1 evening news broadcast on 21 November 1991 (©TVNZ).

Page 96: '... found to be effective against *Staphylococcus aureus*, even when diluted down with water to a concentration of only 1.8% ...'. See Willix, D. et al. (1992).

Page 96: '... *S. aureus* (MRSA) were completely inhibited at 10% honey concentration, a finding that was later confirmed by Rose Cooper, who had begun undertaking pioneering research of her own on manuka honey in Wales.' See Molan, P. (1996) and Cooper, R. et al. (1999).

Page 96: Bill Bracks's recollections of the impact manuka honey had on the fortunes of Comvita were recounted to the author in an interview in December 2013.

Page 97: While the derivation of UMF™ is sometimes disputed, the story recounted here is based on those told to the author in interviews with both Peter Molan and Bill Floyd. The organisation that trademarked it is today called the Unique Manuka Factor Honey Association, and has done outstanding work in protecting the quality image of manuka honey within a very de-regulated marketplace.

Page 100: Stephen Franks's comments about commercial beekeepers are recorded in an article by Stacey Anyan entitled 'The Great Honey Hoo-Ha', which appeared in the April 2010 edition of *North & South* magazine.

Page 102: Bill Floyd wrote a monthly column in the *New Zealand Beekeeping* magazine from 1992 until 2001. The columns detail the many things he and the Marketing Committee were doing to promote New Zealand honey, as well as offering his view on marketing in general, and manuka honey in particular. They provide a fascinating case study on how to improve the image of a commodity food product.

Page 102: For an independent assessment of the growth of the New Zealand honey industry, see *Investment Opportunities in the New Zealand Honey Industry*, produced by the Coriolis Group (2012), and published by *www.foodandbeverage.govt.nz*.

Page 102: Statistics on beekeepers and hive and apiary numbers are published each year by the New Zealand Ministry of Primary Industries.

Page 103: '... it was now seen as "fit for a Queen" ...'. See Vance, A. (2011).

Chapter 5: MERELY A WEED

Page 106: The report on the East Cape forestry scheme, and beekeepers' concerns about its impact on manuka honey production, can be found in the article 'Cape Manuka at Risk' in the December 1992 edition of *Buzzwords*, a National Beekeepers' Association newsletter.

Page 106: John Falloon's quote about manuka being merely a weed was made on New Zealand's public National Radio network on 26 November 1992.

Page 107: There are a number of informative reviews of the sometimes amazing natural history of manuka. Particularly recommended is Derraik, J. (2008) and Stephens, J. and Molan, P. (2005).

Page 107: The ability of manuka to live with its roots submerged for long periods in water is described in detail in Cook, J. et al. (1980).

Page 108: For an interesting discussion on how 'dispersal' has impacted on the development of the New Zealand native ecosystem, see Dawson, M. and Winkworth, R. (2008).

Page 109: As is often the case in botany, you will find various numbers given for the total of *Leptospermum* species in the world. The reference to 88 species used here comes from *The Plant List*, a collaboration between the Royal Botanic Gardens, Kew, and Missouri Botanical Garden (www. theplantlist.org). That would appear to be a fairly authoritative source.

Page 110: '... manuka is the only New Zealand species that releases its seeds during a fire ...'. See Wardle, P. (1991).

Page 111: Joy Thompson's great work (Thompson, 1989), which runs to some 148 pages, is 'A revision of the genus *Leptospermum*', published in the botanical science journal *Telopea*.

Page 112: The case of the cross between a kanuka and a manuka on Great Barrier Island is detailed by Warrick Harris and his colleagues (Harris et al., 1992). Harris is New Zealand's expert in the field, and *Kunzea sinclairii* is the species he says is different from common kanuka.

Page 112: 'A baseline study of what the New Zealand environment was like in 3000 BC ...'. See McGlone, M. (1989).

Page 114: A wonderful book on the many native plants used by Maori, both as implements and as medicines, is Clarke, A. (2007). The description of manuka used to make *korere* can be found on page 226 of that work. Landcare Research in New Zealand also maintains an extensive database on Maori use of native plants.

Page 115: '... there is a theory that kahikatoa means "weapon" ...'. See Stephens, J. and Molan, P. (2005).

Page 115: There are many wonderful books and articles about Joseph Banks and his collections that changed the European world. The statement that the samples he and Solander described increased the number of known species by a quarter comes from Bryson, B. (2003).

Page 116: The sample of manuka Banks and Solander collected at Poverty Bay on 8 October 1769 is *Museum of New Zealand/Te Tongarewa Registration Number SP063724.*

Page 116: 'Solander, for all his great skill in plant classification, incorrectly described both manuka and kanuka as being in the genus *Philadelphus.*' See Harris, W. (1999).

Page 116: 'The Forsters collected samples of manuka at that same tip of the South Island, in Queen Charlotte Sound ...'. See McLintock, A. (1966). The nomenclature, as it appears on the *Flora of New Zealand* website is: Scientific Name: *Leptospermum* J.R. Forst. & G.Forst., Char. Gen. Pl., ed. 2., (1776): Type Taxon: *Leptospermum scoparium* J.R. Forst. & G. Forst.

Page 118: An interesting discussion of Captain Cook's attempts to control scurvy, including the making of beer (as well as the cheeky suggestion that New Zealand's first beer was also a medal-winner) is contained in Kennedy, M. (1996).

Page 118: Details of manuka plants mis-named as a *Philadelphus* being offered for sale in England in 1778 can be found in Harris, W. (1999).

Page 119: An excellent review of the history of manuka cultivation as an ornamental plant is contained in a two-part series by Murray Dawson (Dawson, M., 2009a and 2009b)

Page 119: The names of breeder selections of manuka and other *Leptospermums* come from the Integrated Botanical Information System (IBIS), Australian National Botanic Gardens.

Page 121: Jack Fraser's article in the *New Zealand Journal of Agriculture* is entitled 'Natural and man-made factors limit output of N.Z. honey' (Fraser, J., 1967). The Caterpillar tractor ad is on page 62.

Page 122: 'One commentator insisted that "every plant must be destroyed ..."' See Small, E. (1961).

Page 122: The story of manuka and its blight is presented in van Epenhuijsen, K. et al. (2000).

Page 123: The great authority on New Zealand's many and varied bee species (solitary and otherwise) is Barry Donovan. Barry has spent over 40 years studying solitary bees, has named at least nine new *Leioproctus* species (*L. huakiwi, L. kanapuu, L. keehua, L. otautahi, L. pango, L. waipounamu, L. nunui, L. paahaumaa, L. pekanui*), and was instrumental in the introduction into New Zealand of both leaf-cutter bees and alkali bees for the pollination of lucerne. His magnum opus is Donovan, B. (2007).

Page 127: The observations on possible resource partitioning of honey bees and *Leioproctus* are the author's own, although commercial beekeepers are well aware that their bees collect very little manuka pollen, and few can even tell you what colour the pollen pellets are. I became aware of the different foraging behaviours of the two types of bees when on a number of occasions I took close-up photos of the bees in a large patch of manuka in my back paddock. I have over 1000 pictures of bees working manuka flowers, but in only one of them can you see any manuka pollen on the back legs of honey bees, and even then it is far less than what you would call a purposeful collection. In almost every photograph of *Leioproctus*, on the other hand, they have very large loads of manuka pollen, which is khaki green in colour.

Page 127: A good description of the uses of manuka wood, as well as the reference to those 70-year-old garden tool handles, is Wardle, J. (2011).

Page 127: Details of the use of ti-tree fascines can be found in the historical records of both Morrinsville and the locality of Ohinemuri. The quote that the fascines kept dairy cows from 'disappearing into the mud' comes from 'Early Patetonga Days', a recollection published in the *Ohinemuri Regional History Journal* (McDonald, A., 1974).

Page 127: Pioneering work on manuka oil has been carried out by Nigel Perry and his team at the University of Otago. A review of the properties of the oil is Lis-Balchin, M. et al. (2000).

Page 128: 'New Zealand parrot uses the chewed leaves of manuka to preen itself ...' See Green, T. (1989).

Page 128: The extraction of bio-fuels from manuka on Kawau Island isn't well documented, but some details can be found in 'Yesterdays of Kawau Island' (Holmes, M., 1996), which was published in the island's magazine. The magazine is called *Kookaburra* because Sir George Grey released that Australian bird species on the island in the late nineteenth century.

Page 128: Jonathan Stephens's PhD thesis is available on the University of Waikato website (Stephens, 2006). For a short synopsis, try Stephens, J. and Molan, P. (2008a).

Page 130: Information on the amount of land in manuka/kanuka can be found in the Land Cover Database maintained by the New Zealand Ministry of the Environment. The database figures are on line.

Page 131: The carbon-sequestering abilities of manuka are detailed in Scott, N. et al. (2000).

Page 131: The research programme developing high-performance manuka plantations is a Primary Growth Partnership initiative with commercial partners run in conjunction with the New Zealand Ministry of Primary Industries. Details are available on the MPI website.

Chapter 6: SAVED BY A POT OF HONEY

Page 134: The segment on manuka honey that included the amazing interview with Aaron Phipps appeared on the BBC television programme *Health Check*, 24 August 2000. All quotes are direct transcriptions from that interview.

Page 137: 'Honey — a remedy rediscovered', written by Zumla and Lulat, appeared in the July 1989 issue of the *Journal of the Royal Society of Medicine*.

Page 138: '... we still know more about the structure of the universe than we do about the cells inside us.' See Alberts, B. et al. (2008).

Page 144: Almost every scientific paper on honey and wounds provides a rundown on the various ways honey helps in the healing process. One of the most concise reviews, however, written in Peter Molan's easy-to-understand style, is 'Why honey works well in healing wounds'. It is available on the website Peter has created that includes many of the studies, papers and articles he has written about both manuka honey and woundcare during his long career: www.waikato.academia.edu/PeterMolan/Papers.

Page 145: '... manuka honey with high levels of non-peroxide antibacterial activity (case and clinical studies normally use 12+) can be more effective than honey that only produces hydrogen peroxide ...'. This statement is well supported in the literature, but the most recent comment to that effect comes from Molan, P. (2013).

Page 146: '... Dawn Willix looked at the effect of honey on the seven most common species of bacteria found in wounds.' See Willix, D. et al. (1992).

Page 146: '...found that the same applied to vancomycin-resistant *Enterococci* (VRE).' See Allen, K. et al. (2000).

Page 146: 'The study concluded that this type of manuka honey would prevent the growth of pseudomonas on the surface of a wound ...'. See Cooper, R. and Molan, P. (1999).

Page 148: '... it was the first modern honey-based woundcare product ...'. There are a number of papers that provide details regarding the development of woundcare dressing containing manuka honey. This quote comes from an editorial by Cooper, R. and Jenkins, R. (2012).

Page 150: Julie Betts has written a very concise, peer-reviewed set of woundcare recommendations (Betts, J., 2007), based on her experience using honey on patients in the previous decade. The paper appeared in *Nursing Times*, a leading practitioners' journal in the United Kingdom.

Page 152: Cheryl Dunford's case study report on 'Jem Bonnievale' also appeared in the *Nursing Times* (Dunford, C., 2000). Further case studies using manuka honey were described in a November 2000 article in *Nursing Standard* (Dunford, C. et al, 2000).

Page 153: The BBC *Tomorrow's World* segment where Peter Molan presented his new solid honey dressings (including his entertaining demonstration of where it could be applied) was broadcast on 9 May 2001. The quotes are direct transcriptions taken from that segment.

Page 156: The heart-breaking (and heart-warming) story of the Smith Gate Burns Clinic is told in a series of forms, both in print and on video. Perhaps the best — and the one that shows Ted Fogarty chomping into a manuka honey and alginate dressing — appeared on *Country Morning Today*, a programme produced by the NBC affiliate KFYR-TV in Bismarck, North Dakota. The footage showing the clinic, and interviewing Joe Barzeski, appeared in the United States on the nationwide *CBS Evening News*, 31 July 2008. The quotes that appear here are direct transcriptions taken from those interviews, as well as from a press release from Derma Science on the CBS broadcast dated 4 August 2008.

Page 157: On his waikato.academia.edu website, Peter Molan has kept a record of the honey woundcare products that have been approved around the world (Molan, P., 2012c).

Page 157: The figures on the size of the 'advance wound' treatment market come from a Derma Sciences investor presentation available on the company's website (www.dermasciences.com).

Page 158: A recent summary of honey used in woundcare, including information on the FDA registration of Medihoney, can be found in Lee, D. et al. (2011). In their paper they list six honey woundcare products that have now been approved by the FDA, all but one using manuka honey.

Chapter 7: LET FOOD BE THY MEDICINE

Page 160: The warning by the Acting Director-General of Health appeared in *The New Zealand Herald* on 19 November 1997. It, along with the bee-product label warnings, was the subject of an editorial the author wrote with Ron Law that appeared in *BeeWorld*, the official journal of the International Bee Research Association (Van Eaton, C. and Law, R., 2000).

Page 161: There are numerous books and articles on Hippocrates and his influence on modern medicine. A worthwhile introduction is Scarborough, J. (2002).

Page 163: David Bornstein's comments about the recent development of evidence-based medicine are contained in his 'Fixes' column in the *New York Times* (Bornstein, D., 2012).

Page 165: The review of Cochrane systematic reviews was carried out by El Dib, R. et al. (2007).

Page 166: The most recent review of clinical studies of honey in woundcare is Vandamme, L. et al. (2013). The additional review referred to is Lee, D. et al. (2011).

Page 166: Peter Molan's comments about honey being no more 'alternative' or 'complementary' than other standard wound dressings can be found in Molan, P. (2011).

Page 167: In determining the number of bacterial species that have been shown to be inhibited by honey, the author combined a table drawn up as part of a scientific review of honey he carried out, together with a list Peter Molan has presented in his paper entitled 'The antibacterial activity of honey and its role in treating diseases'. This paper can be found on Peter's website.

Page 168: The first scientific study on the antibacterial activity of honey was Sackett, W. (1919). Contrary to the impression given in the title of the study, Sackett showed that 'the probability of honey acting as a carrier of typhoid fever, dysentery and various diarrhoeal affections is very slight'.

Page 170: The latest review on how manuka honey goes about inhibiting and killing bacteria, including its impact on biofilms, can be found in Maddocks, S. and Jenkins, R. (2013).

Page 170: The comments on the importance of biofilms in human infections comes from the US National Institute of Health (2002).

Page 171: 'Dr Liz Harry and her team at the University of Sydney are doing pioneering work...' See Lu, J. et al. (2014).

Page 171: 'In the time it takes your average human cell to divide just once, a single bacterial cell can make as many as 280,000 *billion* copies of itself ...'. Nobel laureate Christian de Duve, as quoted in Bryson, B. (2003).

Page 171: Perhaps the most up-to-date discussion on the antibacterial properties of honey is Kwakman, P. and Zaat, A. (2012).

Page 172: The comment about bacteria developing resistance to antibiotics faster than we are currently bringing new drugs onto the market comes from Maddocks, S. and Jenkins, R. (2013). The idea that manuka honey working on multiple targets makes it less likely to create resistant bacteria also comes from this paper, one of the most interesting and up-to-date summaries of research on manuka honey you can read anywhere.

Page 172: In the report of their study showing bacteria did not become resistant to manuka honey (Cooper, R. et al, 2010), Rose Cooper and her team reference two papers in relation to bacteria that have become resistant to all known antibiotics, and bacteria that can withstand antiseptics.

Page 173: For an intriguing discussion on the fragility and robustness of systems, natural and otherwise, see Taleb, N. (2012). Taleb contends that both bacteria and our immune system aren't just robust, they are 'anti-fragile'; that is, they are capable of *improving* their ability to overcome problems and shocks over time.

Page 174: The clinical study on the use of honey to treat dehydration in infants suffering from gastroenteritis was Haffejee, I. and Moosa, A. (1985).

Page 175: A report on the laboratory research on manuka honey and *Helicobacter pylori* can be found in Al Somal, N. et al. (1994).

Page 175: The small UK study that didn't find an association between manuka honey and *H. pylori* was published as a short report in the *Journal of the Royal Society of Medicine* (McGovern, D. et al., 1999).

Page 176: For more information on the use of honey in skincare, see Burlando, B. and Cornara, L. (2013).

Page 178: Antifungal activity of honey is described in Brady, N. et al. (1996) and Estevinho, M. et al. (2011).

Page 181: Peter Molan has written excellent summaries on the antioxidant, anti-inflammatory and immuno-stimulatory activities of honey, which can be found on his website. The anti-inflammatory clinical trials, including the one on tonsils and a spoonful of honey (Ozlugedik, S. et al., 2006) are described in detail, along with references to the papers themselves.

Page 182: Amanda Bean's discovery of apalbumin-1 and its increased anti-inflammatory activity in manuka honey was announced in *The New Zealand Beekeeper* (Molan, P., 2012b).

Page 183: The discovery and testing of an arabinogalactan in kanuka honey is described in Gannabathula, S. et al. (2012).

Page 183: There are several good, up-to-date reviews of the therapeutic properties of honey. Highly recommended is Altman, N. (2010). On the internet (bee-hexagon.net) you can also find *The Honey Book*, written by Stefan Bogdanov, a leading expert on honey. Bogdanov's work contains extensive information on the medicinal uses of honey. Both books are very science-based, and include large numbers of references to papers in peer-reviewed journals.

Page 183: The laboratory testing of manuka honey on *Candida* was done by Irish, J. et al. (2006). The clinical trial on pregnant mothers was carried out by Abdelmonem, A. et al. (2012).

Page 183: The testing of manuka honey against species of bacteria causing mastitis in cows was carried out by Allen, K. and Molan, P. (1997). The teat sanitiser that contains manuka honey is Iodoshield Active, manufactured by FIL.

Page 185: Bill Bryson's comments on the number of prescribed drugs that come from plants, and the rather poorer results obtained by combinatorial chemistry can be found on page 325 of *A Short History of Nearly Everything* (2003).

Page 186: Michael Pollan's argument that the antipathy towards natural products as medicines stems from the Church's crusade against paganism can be found in Chapter 2 of his book *The Botany of Desire* (Pollan, M., 2002). The information regarding Paracelsus, the father of pharmacology, appears on page 189 of the book.

Chapter 8: ONE FROM ANOTHER

Page 190: An interesting article describing how hives are taken to Rangitoto Island to produce pohutukawa honey was written by Neil Stuckey of the Waitemata Honey Co. (Stuckey, N., 1994).

Page 192: 'And an important source of information on world honey sources ...'. Crane, E. et al. (1984).

Page 193: European scientists have done considerable work trying to establish protocols for sensory analysis of honey, including a 'lexicon' of honey flavour descriptions, and a set of standards for how honey samples should be assessed. The experiment on the effect of different blends of honey and how they are identified (or mis-identified) by experts comes from a review of the Europeans' work (Piana, M. et al., 2004).

Page 193: There are a number of good reviews of the physico-chemical properties of honey, including White, J. (1975) and White, J. (1992). You will also find good explanations, along with some interesting graphics, in Stefan Bogdanov's *Honey Book*, which is available online. Also recommended is Bogdanov, S. et al. (2004).

Page 193: The study that showed you could transfer thixotropy from heather to clover honey was carried out by Pryce-Jones, and is reported in his 'The rheology of honey' (Pryce-Jones, J., 1936). *Rheology* is the study of the flow of substances, both as liquids and in 'soft-solid' states. Honey is a very interesting and unusual substance in this regard.

Page 195: The classic work on standards for melissopalynology is Louveaux, J. et al. (1978). An excellent hands-on publication on the subject is Sawyer, R. (1988).

Page 196: Anna Maurizio's comments come from 'Microscopy of honey', a chapter she wrote for Eva Crane's *Honey: A Comprehensive Survey* (Maurizio, A., 1975).

Page 196: 'Pollen analysis of manuka honeys', the report by Jonathan Stephens and Peter Molan on non-peroxide activity of manuka honey and pollen content appeared in *The New Zealand Beekeeper* (Stephens, J. and Molan, P., 2008b). Peter is also the author of 'Limitations of the methods of identifying the floral source of honeys', which appeared in *Bee World,* the journal of the International Bee Research Association (Molan, P., 1998).

Page 197: The definitive work on New Zealand pollen is Moar, N. (1993). On page 49 he makes the statement that the pollen of manuka and kanuka cannot be easily separated. He says that, based on the size ranges of the two pollens, 'there may be little difference between them'. Moar's 'Pollen analysis of New Zealand honey', published in the *New Zealand Journal of Agricultural Research* (Moar, N., 1985), recommends 70% manuka pollen as the standard for unifloral honey, but also goes on to say that manuka and kanuka 'produce identical pollen grains'.

Page 197: The comment that in Europe, pollen content is now regarded as a side method comes from Bogdanov, S. (2009).

Page 197: 'As a report from the International Honey Commission points out …'. Oddo, L. and Bogdanov, S. (2004).

Page 198: Peter Molan's statement regarding the finding of the component in manuka honey that gives it its special non-peroxide antibacterial activity is taken from an interview he gave dated 2 February 2013. A video of that interview can be found on the website of Manuka Health (www.manukahealth.co.nz). Peter is being a bit modest, by the way, in saying how long he studied the problem. The first experiment he and Kerry Simpson did was in 1980, and the first announcement of the discovery of the active compound was in a paper that members of the Dresden group presented at a workshop in Naples, Italy, in 2006. So that makes Peter's period of study on the subject about 26 years.

Page 199: Peter Molan outlined the problems and possible solutions to gel diffusion assay testing of manuka honey in an article in *The New Zealand Beekeeper* (Molan, 2008).

Page 200: The famous paper announcing the discovery of MGO as the special non-peroxide activity in manuka honey is Mavric, E. et al. (2008).

Page 200: The University of Waikato paper of that same year is Adams, C. et al. (2008). The paper from Dresden that confirmed the results was Atrott, J. and Henle, T. (2009).

Page 202: The New Zealand study that showed manuka honey with a high non-peroxide activity was safe to eat was Wallace, A. et al. (2009).

Page 202: The Dresden study that showed MGO in manuka honey was broken down by the higher pH present in the lower gut was Degen, J. et al. (2013).

Page 203: The discovery that DHA was responsible for creating MGO in manuka honey was announced in Adams, C. et al. (2009). The discovery was also described in the beekeeping press by the two other members of the Waikato University team. Peter Molan wrote 'Finding how MGO gets to be in manuka honey' in the May 2009 issue of *The New Zealand Beekeeper* (Molan, 2009); Merilyn Manley-Harris was quoted in a press release from the university entitled 'Waikato researchers find source of MGO in active manuka honey' that appeared in the same issue.

Page 203: The paper showing that the DHA/MGO conversion process in manuka honey produces an error in C3/C4 sugar adulteration tests has only recently been accepted for publication. The reference is Rogers, K. et al. (2014).

Page 204: Much of the work of Professor Henle and his team has done in relation to MGO is described on the website of the company Manuka Health (www.manukahealth.co.nz), including a series of informative videos interviewing both Dr Henle and Peter Molan.

Page 204: A handy convertor that allows you to compare MGO amounts and phenol concentration equivalents such as 10+, 15+ and 20+ can be found on the Unique Manuka Factor Honey Association website (www.umf.org.nz).

Page 206: The sensor for fingerprinting red wine is described in Umali, A. et al. (2011). The system is also described on the Royal Society of Chemistry website.

Page 207: 'A recent chemical analysis identified seven such compounds for the first time in manuka honey.' See Oelschlaegel, S. et al. (2012).

Page 207: 'Another phenolic compound called *methyl syringate* has also been found in manuka honey ...'. See Inoue, K. et al. (2005).

Page 207: 'A team lead by Jonathan Stephens also looked at phenolic compounds ...'. See Stephens, J. et al. (2010).

Page 207: The discovery of leptosin is documented in the following two papers: Kato, Y. et al. (2012) and Fearnley, L. et al. (2012).

Epilogue: DISAPPEARING BEES, THE PRICE OF HONEY, AND MAINTAINING A SACRED FLAME

Page 213: '... agricultural production around the world would decrease by about 8%.' See Van Engelsdorp, D. and Meixner, M. (2010).

Page 216: The pollination industry in the United States, as well as the hard lives of commercial beekeepers involved in the trade, is described in detail in Hannah Nordhaus's bestseller, *The Beekeeper's Lament* (Nordhaus, H., 2011).

Page 217: '... especially in California, where over a third of the nation's vegetables and two-thirds of its fruits and nuts are produced.' Source: *California Agricultural Statistics, Crop Year 2012.*

Page 218: For information about varroa, especially in the New Zealand context, see Goodwin, M. and Van Eaton, C. (2001). The book can be read free of charge on the internet at www.biosecurity.govt.nz/files/pests/varroa/control-of-varroa-guide.pdf.

Page 221: The analysis of world beekeeping statistics that shows that, while hive numbers have increased worldwide, they have decreased in the United States and certain parts of Europe, can be found in Van Engelsdorp, D. and Meixner, M. (2010). As for an analysis of world honey production, one study of interest is Aizen, M. and Harder, L. (2009). You can also make your own assessment, however, by going to the statistics website of the Food and Agriculture Organisation of the United Nations (FAOStat: faostat.fao.org). The website is easy to use, and you can learn a lot, not just about world beekeeping, but about all types of agriculture around the globe.

Page 225: The world population at the time this book was written was 7.148 billion. According to *FAOStat*, world honey production in 2012 was 2,044,300 metric tonnes. That is equivalent to a world consumption of 286 grams, or 19 tablespoons per person.

SELECT BIBLIOGRAPHY

Abdelmonem, A. et al. (2012) Bee-honey and yogurt: a novel mixture for treating patients with vulvovaginal candidiasis during pregnancy. *Archives of Gynecology and Obstetrics* 286: 109–114.

Adams, C. et al. (2008) Isolation by HPLC and characterisation of the bioactive fraction of New Zealand manuka honey. *Carbohydrate Research* 343: 651–659.

Adams, C. et al. (2009) The origin of methylglyoxal in New Zealand manuka honey. *Carbohydrate Research* 344: 1050–1053.

Aizen, M. & Harder, L. (2009) The global stock of domesticated honey bees is growing slower than agricultural demand for pollination. *Current Biology* 19: 915–918.

Alberts, B. et al. (2008) *Molecular Biology of the Cell*. 5th ed. New York: Garland Science.

Allen, K. & Molan, P. (1997) The sensitivity of mastitis-causing bacteria to the antibacterial activity of honey. *New Zealand Journal of Agricultural Research* 40: 537–540.

Allen, K. et al. (1991) A survey of the antibacterial activity of some New Zealand honeys. *Journal of Pharmacy and Pharmacology* 43: 817–822.

Allen, K. et al. (2000). The potential for using honey to treat wounds infected with MRSA and VRE. *First World Wound Healing Congress*, Melbourne, Australia.

Allsop, K. & Miller, J. (1996) Honey revisited: a reappraisal of honey in pre-industrial diets. *British Journal of Nutrition* 75: 513–520.

Al Somal, N. et al. (1994) Susceptibility of *H. pylori* to the antibacterial activity of manuka honey. *Journal of the Royal Society of Medicine* 87: 9–12.

Altman, N. (2010) *The Honey Prescription*. Rochester, VT: Healing Arts.

Anonymous (1951) Manuka honey. *The New Zealand Beekeeper* 13(3): 9–28.

Anonymous (1953) Horticulture Division Report. *The New Zealand Beekeeper* 15(6): 33–39.

Anyan, S. (2010) The Great Honey Hoo-Ha. *North & South* 289: 66–74.

Atrott, J. & Henle, T. (2009) Methylglyoxal in manuka honey — correlation with antibacterial properties. *Czech Journal of Food Science* 27: S163–S165.

Avery, B. (2010) *100 Years of Claude Stratford*. Auckland: Lasting Memories.

Bagnall, A. (1982) Heather at Tongariro: a study of a weed introduction. *Tussock Grasslands and Mountainlands Institute Review* 41: 17–21.

Barrett, P. (1995) *The Immigrant Bees 1788 to 1898*. Springwood, NSW: P. Barrett.

Bellamy, D. et al. (1990) *Moa's Ark: The Voyage of New Zealand*. New York: Viking.

Betts, J. (2007) The clinical application of honey in woundcare. *Nursing Times* 104: 43–44.

Bogdanov, S. (2009) Authenticity of honey and other bee products: state of the art. *Bulletin of University of Agricultural Sciences and Veterinary Medicine Cluj-Napoca. Animal Science and Biotechnologies* 64: 1–2.

Bogdanov, S. et al. (2004) Physico-chemical methods for the characterisation of unifloral honey: a review. *Apidologie* 35: S4–S17.

Bornstein, D. (2012) The dawn of the evidence-based budget. *New York Times*, 30 May, page 13.

Brady, N. et al. (1996) The sensitivity of dermatophytes to the antimicrobial activity of manuka honey and other honey. *Pharmaceutical Sciences* 2: 471–473.

Bryson, B. (2003) *A Short History of Nearly Everything*. London: Doubleday.

Bryson, B. (2010*) At Home*. London: Doubleday.

Burlando, B. & Cornara, L. (2013) Honey in dermatology and skin care: a review. *Journal of Cosmetic Dermatology* 12: 306–313.

Caron, D. et al. (2013) *Honey Bee Biology and Beekeeping*, rev. ed. Kalamazoo, MI: Wicwas.

Clarke, A. (2007). *The Great Sacred Forest of Tane*. Auckland: Reed.

Cook, J. et al. (1980) Responses of *Leptospermum scoparium* and *L. ericoides* to waterlogging. *New Zealand Journal of Botany* 18: 233–246.

Cooper, R. & Jenkins, R. (2012) Are there feasible prospects for manuka honey as an alternative to conventional antimicrobial? *Expert Review of Anti-Infective Therapy* 10: 623–625.

Cooper, R. & Molan, P. (1999). The use of honey as an antiseptic in managing *Pseudomonas* infection. *Journal of Wound Care* 8: 161–164.

Cooper, R. et al. (1999) Antibacterial activity of honey against strains of *Staphylococcus aureus* from infected wounds. *Journal of the Royal Society of Medicine* 92: 283–285.

Cooper, R. et al. (2010) Absence of bacterial resistance to medical-grade manuka honey. *European Journal of Clinical Microbiology and Infectious Diseases* 29: 1237–1241.

Coriolis Group (2012) *Investment Opportunities in the New Zealand Honey Industry*. Wellington: Ministry of Economic Development.

Crane, E., ed. (1975) *Honey: A Comprehensive Survey*. London: Heinemann.

Crane, E. (1980) *A Book of Honey*. Oxford: Oxford University Press.

Crane, E. (1983) *The Archaeology of Beekeeping*. London: Duckworth.

Crane, E. (1999) *The World History of Beekeeping and Honey Hunting*. London: Duckworth.

Crane, E. et al. (1984) *Directory of Important World Honey Sources*. Gerrards Cross: International Bee Research Association.

Dawson, C. (1979) Waitangi Treaty had links with first beekeeper. *The New Zealand Beekeeper* 40(1): 19–22.

Dawson, M. (2009a) A history of *Leptospermum scoparium* in cultivation 1) discoveries from the wild. *The New Plantsman* 4: 51–59.

Dawson, M. (2009b) A history of *Leptospermum scoparium* in cultivation 2) garden selections. *The New Plantsman* 4: 67–78.

Dawson, M. & Winkworth, R. (2008) The New Zealand flora: 'Moa's Ark' or 'fly-paper of the Pacific'? *New Zealand Garden Journal* 11: 20–24.

Degen, J. et al. (2013) Metabolic transit of dietary methylglyoxal. *Journal of Agricultural and Food Chemistry* 61: 10253–10260.

Derraik, J. (2008) New Zealand manuka: a brief account of its natural history and human perceptions. *New Zealand Garden Journal* 11: 4–8.

Donovan, B. (2007) *Apoidea: Fauna of New Zealand, No. 57*. Lincoln: Manaaki Whenua Press, Landcare Research.

Dunford, C. (2000). Using honey as a dressing for infected skin lesions. *Nursing Times* 96: 7–9.

Dunford, C. et al. (2000). The use of honey in wound management. *Nursing Standard* 15: 63–68.

El Dib, R. et al. (2007) Mapping the Cochrane evidence for decision making in health care. *Journal of Evaluation in Clinical Practice* 13: 689–692.

Estevinho, M. et al. (2011) Antifungal effect of lavender honey against *Candida albicans*, *C. krusei* and *Cryptococcus neoformans*. *Journal of Food Science and Technology* 48: 640–643.

Fearnley, L. et al. (2012) Compositional analysis of manuka honeys by high-resolution mass spectrometry: identification of a manuka-enriched archetypal molecule. *Food Chemistry* 132: 948–953.

Floyd, B. (1991) Honey, sweeter than wine ... *The New Zealand Beekeeper* 211: 14–19.

Fraser, J. (1967) Natural and man-made factors limit output of N.Z. honey. *New Zealand Journal of Agriculture* 115: 57–63.

Gannabathula, S. et al. (2012) Arabinogalactan proteins contribute to the immunostimulatory properties of New Zealand honeys. *Immunopharmacology and Immunotoxicology* 34: 598–607.

Goodwin, M. & Van Eaton, C. (1999) *Control of American Foulbrood Without the Use of Drugs*. Wellington: National Beekeepers' Association of New Zealand.

Goodwin, M. & Van Eaton, C. (2001). *Control of Varroa — A Guide for New Zealand Beekeepers*. Wellington: New Zealand Ministry of Agriculture and Forestry.

Graham, J., ed. (1992) *The Hive and the Honey Bee*. Hamilton, IL: Dadant & Sons.

Great Barrier Island Charitable Trust (2010). Chapter 9: Vegetation, *Great Barrier Island (Aotea) State of Environment Report*. Auckland: Great Barrier Island Charitable Trust.

Green, T. (1989) Antiparasitic behaviour in New Zealand parakeets. *Notornis* 36: 322–323.

Haffejee, I. & Moosa, A. (1985) Honey in the treatment of infantile gastroenteritis. *British Medical Journal* 290: 1866.

Haines, M. (1975) Handling manuka honey: part II. *The New Zealand Beekeeper* 37(3): 62–63.

Harris, W. (1999). The domestication of New Zealand plants. *Proceedings, New Zealand Plants and Their Story Conference*. Wellington, October 1999, pages 1–3.

Harris, W. et al. (1992). Observations on biosystematic relationships of *Kunzea sinclairii* and on an intergeneric hybrid *Kunzea sinclairii × Leptospermum scoparium*. *New Zealand Journal of Botany* 30: 213–230.

Holmes, M. (1996) Yesterdays of Kawau Island. *Kookaburra*. Spring: 46–53.

Honey Marketing Authority (1967) Does our future lie in retail packs or bulk selling? *The New Zealand Beekeeper* 29(2): 14–19.

Hopkins, I. (1886) *The Illustrated Australasian Bee Manual and Complete Guide to Modern Bee Culture in the Southern Hemisphere,* 3rd ed. Auckland: I. Hopkins.

Hopkins, I. (1926) *Practical Beekeeping*. Auckland: Whitcombe and Tombs.

Hornsey, I. (2003) *A History of Beer and Brewing*. Cambridge: Royal Society of Chemistry.

Horticulture Division. (1951) Address by Director. *The New Zealand Beekeeper* 13(3): 24–25.

Inoue, K. et al. (2005) Identification of phenolic compound in manuka honey as specific superoxide anion radical scavenger using electron spin resonance (ESR) and liquid chromatography with coulometric array detection. *Journal of Science of Food and Agriculture* 85: 872–878.

Irish, J. et al. (2006) Honey has an antifungal effect against *Candida* species. *Medical Mycology* 44: 289–291.

Kato, Y. et al. (2012) Identification of a novel glycoside, leptosin, as a chemical marker of manuka honey. *Journal of Agricultural and Food Chemistry* 60: 3418–3423.

Kennedy, M. (1996) Biotechnology brought to New Zealand by Captain James Cook aboard the *Endeavour, Resolution, Adventure* and *Discovery*. *Australasian Biotechnology* 6: 156–160.

Kwakman, P. & Zaat, A. (2012) Antibacterial components of honey: a critical review. *IUBMB Life* 64: 48–55.

Lee, D. et al. (2011) Honey and wound healing: an overview. *American Journal of Dermatology* 12: 181–190.

Lennon, W. (1948) *Bees in Their Bonnets*. Timaru: Benyon.

Lévi-Strauss, C. (1974) *From Honey to Ashes*. New York: Harper and Row.

Lis-Balchin, M. et al. (2000) Pharmacological and antimicrobial studies on different tea tree oils originating in Australia and New Zealand. *Phytotherapy Research* 14: 623–629.

Louveaux, J. et al. (1978) Methods of Melissopalynology. *Bee World* 59: 139–157.

Low, T. (1989) *Bush Tucker — Australia's Wild Food Harvest*. North Ryde, NSW: Angus & Robertson.

Lu, J. et al. (2014) Manuka-type honeys can eradicate biofilms produced by *Staphylococcus aureus* strains with different biofilm-forming abilities. *PeerJ* 2: e326.

Maddocks, S. & Jenkins, R. (2013) Honey: a sweet solution to the growing problem of antimicrobial resistance? *Future Microbiology* 8: 1419–1429.

Matheson, A. & Reid, M. (2011) *Practical Beekeeping in New Zealand*, 4th ed. Auckland: Exisle.

Maurizio, A. (1975) Chapter 7: Microscopy of honey. In Crane, E., ed. *Honey: A Comprehensive Survey*. London: Heinemann.

Mavric, E. et al. (2008). Identification and quantification of methylglyoxal as the dominant antibacterial constituent of Manuka honeys from New Zealand. *Molecular Nutrition and Food Research* 52: 483–489.

McDonald, A. (1974) Early Patetonga days. *Ohinemuri Regional History Journal* 18: 35–36.

McDonough, W. & Braungart, M. (2002) *Cradle to Cradle*. New York: North Point.

McGlone, M. (1989) The Polynesian settlement of New Zealand in relation to environmental and biotic changes. *New Zealand Journal of Ecology* 12: 115–129.

McGovern, D. et al. (1999) Manuka honey against *H. pylori. Journal of the Royal Society of Medicine* 92: 439.

McLintock, A., ed. (1966) The Cook era. *An Encyclopedia of New Zealand*. Wellington: Government Press.

Michner, C. (1974) *The Social Behaviour of Bees*. Cambridge, MA: Harvard University Press.

Moar, N. (1985) Pollen analysis of New Zealand honey. *New Zealand Journal of Agricultural Research* 28: 39–70.

Moar, N. (1993) *Pollen Grains of New Zealand Dicotyledonous Plants*. Lincoln: Manaaki Whenua Press, Landcare Research.

Molan, P. (1996) Honey as an antimicrobial agent. In Mizrahi, A. & Lensky, Y., eds. *Bee Products: Properties, Applications and Apitherapy*. New York: Plenum, pages 27–37.

Molan, P. (1998) Limitations of the methods of identifying the floral source of honeys. *Bee World* 79: 59–68.

Molan, P. (1999) The role of honey in the management of wounds. *Journal of Wound Care* 8: 423–426.

Molan, P. (2000) Selection of honey for use as a wound dressing. *Primary Intention (The Australian Journal of Wound Management)* 8: 87–92.

Molan, P. (2001) Potential of honey for the treatment of wounds and burns. *American Journal of Clinical Dermatology* 2: 13–19.

Molan, P. (2002) Re-introducing honey in the management of wounds and ulcers — theory and practice. *Ostomy/Wound Management* 48: 28–40.

Molan, P. (2006) The evidence supporting the use of honey as a wound dressing. *International Journal of Lower Extremity Wounds* 5: 40–54.

Molan, P. (2008) Improvements to the UMF assay. *New Zealand Beekeeper* 16(7): 24–25.

Molan, P. (2009) Finding how MGO gets to be in manuka honey. *The New Zealand Beekeeper* 17(4): 16.

Molan, P. (2011) The evidence and rationale for the use of honey as a wound dressing. *Wound Practice and Research* 19: 204–220.

Molan, P. (2012a) What's special about active manuka honey. http://waikato.academia.edu/PeterMolan.

Molan, P. (2012b) Honey anti-inflammatory factor identified. *The New Zealand Beekeeper* 20(8): 6.

Molan, P. (2012c) Honey wound-care products available as registered medical devices. http://waikato.academia.edu/PeterMolan.

Molan, P. (2013) The use of manuka honey to promote wound healing. *L.O.G.I.C., The Official Journal of the New Zealand College of Primary Health Care Nurses* 12: 23–25.

Molan, P. & Betts, J. (2000) Using honey as a wound dressing: some practical considerations. *Nursing Times* 96: 36–37.

Molan, P. & Betts, J. (2004) Clinical usage of honey as a wound dressing: an update. *Journal of Wound Care* 13: 353–358.

Molan, P. & Betts, J. (2008) Using honey to heal diabetic foot ulcers. *Advances in Skin and Wound Care* 21: 313–316.

Molan, P. & Russell, K. (1988) Non-peroxide antibacterial activity in some New Zealand honeys. *Journal of Apicultural Research* 27: 62–67.

Molan, P. et al. (1988) A comparison of the antibacterial activities of some New Zealand honeys. *Journal of Apicultural Research* 27: 252–256.

Morales, G. et al. (1988) Life history of the sooty beech scale (*Ultracoelostoma assimile*) in New Zealand *Nothofagus* forests. *New Zealand Entomologist* 11: 24–37.

Nelson, R. (2003) Antibiotic development pipeline runs dry — new drugs to fight resistant organisms are not being developed, experts say. *The Lancet* 362: 1726–1727.

Nordhaus, H. (2011) *The Beekeeper's Lament*. New York: Harper Perennial.

Oddo, L. & Bogdanov, S. (2004) Determination of honey botanical origin: problems and issues. *Apidologie* 35: S2–S3.

Oelschlaegel, S. et al. (2012) Classification and characterization of manuka honeys based on phenolic compounds and methylglyoxal. *Journal of Agricultural and Food Chemistry* 60: 7229–7237.

'On The Land'. (1910) Bush versus clover honey. *The New Zealand Herald.* XLVII: 8 (10 March).

Ozlugedik, S. et al. (2006) Can postoperative pains following tonsillectomy be relieved by honey? A prospective, randomized, placebo controlled preliminary study. *International Journal of Pediatric Otorhinolaryngology* 70: 1929–1934.

Piana, M. et al. (2004). Sensory analysis applied to honey: state of the art. *Apidologie* 35: S26–S37.

Pollan, M. (2002) *The Botany of Desire*. New York: Random House.

Pollan, M. (2006) *The Omnivore's Dilemma*. New York: Penguin.

Pollan, M. (2013) *Cooked: A Natural History of Transformation*. New York: Penguin.

Poupard, J. et al. (1994) The evolution of antimicrobial susceptibility testing methods. In Poupard, J. et al., eds. *Antimicrobial Susceptibility Testing.* New York: Plenum, pages 3–14.

Pryce-Jones, J. (1936) The rheology of honey. In Scott Blair, G., ed. *Foodstuffs: Their Plasticity, Fluidity and Consistency.* Amsterdam: N. Holland.

Riley, J. et al. (2005) The flight paths of honeybees recruited by the waggle dance. *Nature* 435: 205–207.

Rogers, K. et al. (2014) The unique manuka effect: why New Zealand manuka honey fails the AOAC 998.12 C-4 sugar method — Part 2. *Journal of Agricultural and Food Chemistry,* 62:2615-22. Pre-publication.

Russell, K. (1983) The antibacterial activities of honey. Unpublished MSc thesis. Hamilton, NZ: University of Waikato.

Sackett, W. (1919) *Honey as a Carrier of Intestinal Diseases*. Bulletin of the Colorado State University Agricultural Experimental Station No. 252.

Sawyer, R. (1988) *Honey Identification*. Cardiff: Cardiff Academic Press.

Scarborough, J. (2002) Hippocrates and the Hippocratic Ideal in modern medicine: a review essay of *Hippocrates* by Jaques Jouanna. *International Journal of the Classical Tradition* 9: 287–297.

Scott, N. et al. (2000) Carbon and nitrogen distribution and accumulation in a New Zealand scrubland ecosystem. *Canadian Journal of Forest Research*. 30: 1246–1255.

Seeley, T. (2009) *The Wisdom of The Hive: The Social Physiology of Honey Bee Colonies*. Cambridge, MA: Harvard University Press.

Simone-Finstrom, M. & Spivak, M. (2012) Increased resin collection after parasite challenge: a case of self-medication in honey bees? *PLOS ONE* 7: e34601.

Small, E. (1961) The problems of undeveloped hill country with particular reference to the east coast. *Sheepfarming Annual* 14: 67–69.

Stephens, J. (2006) The factors responsible for the varying levels of UMF® in manuka (*Leptospermum scoparium*) honey. Unpublished PhD thesis. Hamilton, NZ: University of Waikato.

Stephens, J. & Molan, P. (2005) A review of *Leptospermum scoparium* in New Zealand. *New Zealand Journal of Botany* 43: 431–449.

Stephens, J. & Molan, P. (2008a) The explanation of why the level of UMF varies in manuka honey. *The New Zealand Beekeeper* 16(3): 11–13.

Stephens, J. & Molan, P. (2008b). Pollen analysis of manuka (*Leptospermum scoparium*) honeys. *The New Zealand Beekeeper* 16(8): 8–12.

Stephens, J. et al. (2010) Phenolic compounds and methylglyoxal in some New Zealand manuka and kanuka honeys. *Food Chemistry* 120: 78–86.

Stuckey, N. (1994). The joys of keeping bees on an island. *The New Zealand Beekeeper* 1(2): 1.

Taleb, N. (2012) *Antifragile: Things That Gain from Disorder*. New York: Random House.

Tan, S. et al. (1988) Extractives from New Zealand honeys 1. white clover, manuka and kanuka unifloral honeys. *Journal of Agricultural and Food Chemistry* 36: 453–460.

Taylor, R. (1868) *The Past and Present of New Zealand*. London: William Macintosh.

Thompson, J. (1989) A revision of the genus *Leptospermum*. *Telopea* 3: 301–448.

Umali, A. et al. (2011) Discrimination of flavonoids and red wine varietals by arrays of differential peptidic sensors. *Journal of the Royal Society of Chemistry* 2: 439–445.

US National Institute of Health (2002). *Research on Microbial Biofilms*. Bethesda, MY: USNIH.

Van Eaton, C. & Law, R. (2000) Marketing apitherapy products and the challenge of government regulation. *BeeWorld* 82: 109–115.

Van Engelsdorp, D. & Meixner, M. (2010) A historical review of managed honey bee populations in Europe and the United States and the factors that may affect them. *Journal of Invertebrate Pathology* 103: S80–S95.

van Epenhuijsen, K. et al. (2000) The rise and fall of manuka blight scale: a review of the distribution of *Eriococcus orariensis* in New Zealand. *New Zealand Entomologist* 23: 67–70.

van Ketel, B. (1892) Festnummer der Berichten van den Niederlandsche Maatschappij. *Bevordering der Pharmacie* 67: 96; as reported in Dustmann, J. (1979) Antibacterial effect of honey. *Apiacta* 14: 7–11.

Vance, A. (2011) Tea and manuka honey a Kiwi treat fit for a Queen. *Fairfax NZ News*, 27 April.

Vandamme, L. et al. (2013) Honey in modern wound care: a systematic review. *Burns* 39: 1514–1525.

Wacey, D. et al. (2011) Microfossils of sulphur-metabolizing cells in 3.4-billion-year-old rocks of Western Australia. *Nature Geoscience* 4: 698–702.

Wallace, A. et al. (2009) Demonstrating the safety of manuka honey UMF® 20+ in a human trial with healthy individuals. *British Journal of Nutrition* 103: 1023–1028.

Ward, A. (1986) Honey changes may mean marketing authority answers. *The Agricultural Economist* 7: 25–28.

Wardle, J. (2011) *Wardle's Native Trees of New Zealand.* Wellington: New Zealand Farm Forestry Association.

Wardle, P. (1991) *Vegetation of New Zealand.* Caldwell, NJ: Blackburn.

White, J. (1975) Chapter 5: Composition of honey; Chapter 6: Physical characteristics of honey. In Crane, E., ed. *Honey: A Comprehensive Survey.* London: Heinemann.

White, J. (1992) Chapter 21: Honey. In Graham, J., ed. *The Hive and the Honey Bee.* Hamilton, IL: Dadant & Sons.

Wilkinson, E. et al. (1979) *Thyme in Central Otago.* Lincoln, NZ: Tussock Grasslands and Mountainlands Institute.

Willix, D. et al. (1992) A comparison of the sensitivity of wound-infecting species of bacteria to the antibacterial activity of manuka honey and other honey. *Journal of Applied Bacteriology* 73: 388–394.

Winston, M. (1987) *The Biology of the Honey Bee.* Cambridge, MA: Harvard University Press.

Winter, T. (1962) *Beekeeping in New Zealand.* Wellington: New Zealand Department of Agriculture.

Yang, S. (1998) *The Divine Farmer's Materia Medica: A Translation of the Shen Nong Ben Cao Jing.* Boulder, CO: Blue Poppy.

Zumla, A. & Lulat, A. (1989). Honey — a remedy rediscovered. *Journal of the Royal Society of Medicine* 82: 384.

INDEX

enquiry 167–9; systematic reviews
164–5
exports 102; deregulation 81; export
controls 70–9; export licensing 71;
exporting package bees 79; free-
trade 81; grade standards 72–3,
191–4; stamp duty, honey seals 72
extracting honey 58, 75–6; Norwegian
'Honningløsner' (honey-loosener)
75, 76

Falloon, John 106
Federal Drug Administration (FDA)
gold standard 158, 184
Feminine Monarchie, The 51–2
fermentation 40–1, 43–4, 45–7, 50,
117–18; bee bread 43–4
fishing and hunting implements 114
Fleming, Alexander 16–17
Floyd, Bill 84, 89, 95, 101, 148, 174,
175
Floyd, Sandee 92
Fogarty, Ted 154, 155
Food and Agriculture Organisation
(UN) 190
Forster, George 116
Forster, J R 116
foulbrood control 67–8, 87
Franks, Stephen 100
Fraser, Jack 120
free trade 81
fructose 41–2, 193

garden implements and fencing 114,
127
giant honey bee (*Apis dorsata*) 33, 49
Gibbs, Robert 69
Gittos, Mrs 63
gluconic acid 24, 41
glucose 41–2, 57, 193
glucose oxidase 41–2, 142, 168
Good Manufacturing Practice (GMP)
system: wound dressings 151
Government Apiarist 66–9, 77
Great Barrier Island 56–9
Greek influences 47–8

Haines, Bill 78
Haines, Malcolm 78–9
Harry, Liz 171
harvesting honey: history 30–3, 49;
honey hunters 30–2, 33
healing with honey 141–6, 153–4,
167–71, 178; antibacterial effect

142–3; antifungal properties
177–8; antioxidant activities
178–81; debrider of dead tissue
142; deodorising wounds 142;
eradication of biofilms 169–71;
immune-stimulatory effect 182;
interference with bacteria's gene
regulation 171; moisturising
properties 141, 144–5, 181;
prebiotic properties 183; protection
from bacteria 141; reduction in
adhesins 170; respiratory burst
to destroy bacteria 142; tissue
regrowth 178
health warnings 159
heather (*Calluna vulgaris*) 21
Henle, Thomas 198, 200–2
Hinduism (Rig Veda 1) 46
Hippocrates 48, 160–3, 186
Hippocratic oath 162
hive levy 101
hive locations 102–3, 130
hive numbers 220–4
hive tool 45
hives: foundation press 58, 66; frames
56; moveable frame hives 52–3, 66;
skeps 53, 54, 66–9; supers 56
HMS *Endeavour* 105, 115
HMS *Resolution* 116
hobbyists 99
Hobson, Lieutenant Governor William
61, 65
holistic approach to medicine 162
Holland's brand 81
honesty box sales 78
honey bees 30–55, 210–25; anatomy
38–9; castes 35; colony collapse
disorder 211–12; communication
between 35; disappearing honey
bees meme 210–24; drones 34, 35;
honey ripening 39–42; insecticides
211; introduction to Australia 64;
introduction to New Zealand 62,
65; nectar gathering 38–9; pollen
collection 42–4; propolis 45;
queen bees 33–5; relationship with
humans 30–6, 45; relationship with
plants 37; resin collection 44–5;
self-medication 44–5; species of
bees 33, 49; stages of honey bee
brood 43; sustainable bi-vores 36–
7; varroa parasite 99, 211, 217–22;
weather conditions 69, 100; worker
bees 33–4, 35